CW00538648

Justin Derwent grew up in Yorkshire and qualified in dentistry at Leeds University. Later he studied for a Master's degree in medical law at Cardiff University. He now lives with his wife and their ever-increasing family of animals in an old farmhouse on the Dorset/Somerset border.

PRACTICE MAKES PERFECT

To Chloe, my little Yorkshire terrier who sat on my lap
for many hours whilst I wrote this book.

Justin Derwent

PRACTICE MAKES PERFECT

AUSTIN MACAULEY
PUBLISHERS LTD.

A CIP catalogue record for this title is available from the British Library.

ISBN 9781849633215

www.austinmacauley.com

First Published (2013)
Austin Macauley Publishers Ltd.
25 Canada Square
Canary Wharf
London
E14 5LB

Printed & Bound in Great Britain

CHAPTER ONE

I cannot ever recall feeling more undecided about anything. Admittedly I was struggling to make the right decision on the sort of situation which is encountered only occasionally in life, and it was undoubtedly one of the most important decisions I would ever have to make. I knew that whatever I decided would probably determine the path the rest of my life would take. This was a frightening thought and in the circumstances, perhaps it was understandable that I could not see a clear way ahead. My mother always said that Librans are very indecisive so perhaps my birth sign was to blame. Whatever the reason, I was finding it impossible to make up my mind.

My university career was finally behind me and here I was, a newly qualified dental surgeon, standing at a crossroads in my life. I had to decide now whether to stay on at the dental hospital and follow an academic career or make the break and branch out into general practice. When I first became a student, there had never been any doubt about it; I had gone to study dentistry in order to become an ordinary general practice dentist. At the time, the whole thing had been clear in my mind. I had a specific target and I aimed for it. In fact, being so certain about it had helped me to get through the years of study. As my course progressed, however, my feelings on the subject altered somewhat. I discovered that I was quite good at passing exams and many of my tutors expressed the opinion that I would probably be suited to an academic career. The more I thought about it the more attractive the idea became. I would remain at the hospital, which had now become familiar ground, and I felt relatively safe and comfortable there. But, it would be a long, slow haul before I reached a position of any standing, and there would be little financial reward in the early days. Perhaps my real reason for wanting to stay on at the hospital was that I had been very happy as a student and it was natural to try and cling on to the happiness I had found over the past few years.

On the other hand, general practice would bring new challenges. I would have status and independence right from the start and earn much more money. I definitely needed money. Living on a grant for such a long time had caused me to run up a considerable overdraft. The bank manager would now be looking to me to clear it. It would also be nice to be able to buy clothes, eat out in restaurants, and go away on holiday. There were so many things I wanted; things I had not even been able to think about as a student. General practice would revolutionise my life in this respect.

I had asked the Dean for his advice, and he was in absolutely no doubt at all as to what I should do.

'You'll be a bloody fool if you go into general practice', came his blunt reply. 'Look at me,' he went on. 'I do very little now except sit back and take responsibility, and I'm paid a big fat salary. It's true that you won't be paid much to start with if you stay on at the hospital but your salary will steadily increase over the years and, in the end, you'll be very comfortably off. You might be able to earn big money from the start in general practice but as you get older you'll find it difficult to keep up the pace. However, if you slow down, your earnings will diminish. Unfortunately, you'll have become accustomed to a particular lifestyle and you won't readily accept a drop in income. In the end you'll kill yourself trying to maintain your standard of living.'

'But I'm desperately short of money,' I protested. 'Perhaps I could do a year or two in general practice to get myself on my feet financially, then come back to the hospital.'

'That sounds a good idea now, but the truth is, you'll be very reluctant to take a drop in salary at the hospital, having had a taste of what you can earn in general practice. In fact, you may not be able to. I've seen it all before. Students leave here and find they can earn big money in general practice if they're prepared to work hard. What they fail to realise is that it doesn't all belong to them. The taxman will demand a large proportion of it as soon as he catches up with them. Unfortunately, by the time the tax demand arrives, they've spent everything they've earnt, so then they have to work even harder to pay off the tax bill. At the same time. They've invariably been tempted into a mortgage on some luxurious bachelor flat or taken on hire purchase commitments to buy a flashy car or boat. After a couple of years, they're so deeply submersed in this financial quagmire they can't even begin to contemplate a drop in salary, so any thoughts they might have had about returning to a hospital career have to be abandoned.

'Also, you may well find that after a few years, general practice dentistry becomes rather boring and you won't get much opportunity to discuss your ideas and experiences with people of a similar intellect as yourself. You have shown yourself capable of passing exams without too much difficulty, and I would say that you are ideally suited to an academic career. If I were you I would give up all thoughts of general practice and get started on studying for higher qualifications as soon as possible.'

It was sound advice and he could not have been more positive that it was the right course of action for me. Why then was I, at this moment, sitting on a train heading south for the purpose of going to an interview for a position in general practice?

I had seen the advertisement in the British Dental Journal and for some reason I had been very strongly tempted to apply for the post. It was for an associate dental surgeon in the attractive little town of Luccombury in the most unspoilt and picturesque part of Dorset. For the past two weeks I had been thinking about it. I knew from my pre-university days when I had lived on the south coast, that southern winters were much milder than in the north. There was less fog, rain and snow and everything was much cleaner with less pollution. Luccombury seemed an ideal place to live.

Finally, one evening, some strange driving force made me write a reply to the advertisement. I decided that I ought at least go along to see the practice, meet the principal and find out how I felt about the town, the practice and the prospect of moving south. Perhaps my feelings would be different when the prospect became a reality rather than something based on memories and imagination. I was also a great believer in fate. It seemed to me, from my limited experience of life, that if something was meant to be, it just tended to happen without a lot of effort going into it. I believed that if one had to struggle to bring about a change in one's life, it probably wasn't really the right way to go.

A reply to my letter came back very quickly inviting me to attend for interview, and now here I was on my way there. Throughout the train journey, I had considered over and over again the arguments for and against a career in general practice dentistry. I knew that the Dean's advice made a lot of sense and that, if I were honest, the reasons for staying on at the hospital probably outweighed those for leaving. My mind was literally buzzing with it all, but as the miles rolled by, I became increasingly aware that I wanted new challenges and independence. I was looking for a different life and a change of environment. I had enjoyed my time at the dental hospital but I was beginning to feel that now I was probably ready to move on.

I was so deeply immersed in my thoughts that I nearly missed my station. I suddenly realised that the train was standing still and I was looking out of the window at the sign for Sonnington. I leapt to my feet, snatched my suitcase from the luggage rack and just managed to get off the train before it drew away again.

From Sonnington I had to take a bus. Surprisingly, I did not have long to wait for one and some thirty minutes later I was in the market square in the centre of the quaint little town of Luccombury. It was exactly as I remembered it though it was at least seven years since my last visit. For a small town it had more than its fair share of inns and public houses each with ornate signs, welcoming stone entrance porches and stone mullioned windows. The autumn sun was low in the sky and cast a golden yellow light over the streets and rooftops. From the shop windows, amber reflections flashed back at me as I strolled along. The reds, browns and yellows of the trees in and around the town provided focal points of colour, which contrasted with the relatively monochromatic buff-toned buildings. It was a particularly attractive time of the year and I had arrived there to witness its full splendour. Everything was exactly like the mental picture I had carried with me, but I was particularly struck with how very different it was from the austere streets of the northern city around the dental hospital. It was all so clean, bright and colourful by comparison. If any forces were at play trying to influence my decision they were certainly setting a most attractive and tempting scene in Luccombury that day.

CHAPTER TWO

I wasn't the slightest bit apprehensive as I arrived at the gate of the large seventeenth century house I was looking for. As I wasn't sure whether or not I wanted the job, I decided that the best course of action was simply to play it by ear and see how things turned out.

I was immediately impressed by the gleaming brass practice nameplate at the side of the door indicating that I was standing outside the surgery of 'Mr Spencer Padginton LDSRCS (Eng), Dental Surgeon'. Alongside it was a sign announcing that the building was named 'Fothergill House'. For a moment I tried to visualise my own name followed by my newly acquired qualifications on a similar plate fixed to the Hamstone wall. I hadn't thought about brass nameplates before. In some ways it seemed a bit ostentatious to display one's qualifications and professional status to everyone who passed by. On the other hand, it was something to be proud of and why shouldn't one advertise oneself in this way? Thousands of other people do it – doctors, solicitors, accountants, vets. After all, its real purpose was to attract clients, or in this case, patients; it wasn't just to show off. It then occurred to me that I wouldn't have a brass nameplate if I stayed on at the hospital. Did that really matter? Of course it didn't. It was certainly not important enough to influence my decision about the future.

A sign at the other side of the heavy, cream-painted front door invited patients visiting the practice to ring and enter, so I pressed the shiny brass bell and pushed the door open.

The familiar smell of antiseptic mixed with oil of cloves greeted me. Although I was, by now, quite accustomed to what was simply the characteristic smell of a dental surgery, I thought it seemed particularly strong and I felt sure that it must seem very powerful indeed to patients.

I entered the spacious entrance hall, which immediately created a good impression, due mainly to the highly polished antique oak sideboard and the oak desk, which seemed to me to be quality pieces of furniture. The decor, however, was not spectacular; the low ceiling did not help to hide the fact that the paint on the upper parts of the walls was very discoloured and, in places was flaking quite badly. The walls were painted dove grey and the woodwork cream, and although the choice of colours was uninspiring, the polished oak floors with scattered rugs enhanced the overall effect. There were gleaming ornate brass finger plates on the doors, which immediately caught the eye, though I imagine that strictly speaking they were of a different era from the rest of the house. On the left was a door marked 'waiting room' and the staircase ran up the opposite wall.

I did not have long to wait before a figure appeared at the top of the stairs. He was about forty-five years old and to describe him as portly would have been a bit unkind. Let us just say he looked as if he was the sort of person who enjoyed his food. He had a round, open face and short dark hair. He was wearing a bright red T-shirt bearing the name 'Alfa Romeo', an old pair of shapeless brown corduroy trousers and an equally old pair of oily brown suede shoes. He was smoking a pipe.

'Hello, there,' he shouted cheerily. 'You must be Mr Derwent.'

'That's right, Justin Derwent. I'm here about the vacancy.'

'Spencer Padginton. How do you do? Thanks for coming, Justin. Did you have a good journey?' He shook my hand warmly.

'Yes thank you, not bad at all. It didn't take as long as I thought it would. I'm actually a bit early, I hope it isn't inconvenient for you.'

'Not at all, my dear chap. I wasn't expecting you just yet or I would have changed. I've been working on one of my cars. But it doesn't matter that you are early; I'm delighted to see you. Please come in and sit down, and I'll get you a drink.'

He led the way through the door at the bottom of the stairs into a large, comfortable sitting room. Quite clearly, this room had not been decorated for many years but there was an aura of quality about it in spite of the yellowing white paint and numerous scuffmarks around the skirting board.

'Take a seat. Can I get you a beer?'

'Yes, thank you; that would be very welcome. It's quite warm today.'

'It's surprisingly warm for the time of year. It's come as quite a change after all the rain we had last week, but that's English weather, isn't it?'

He filled two glasses with a slightly cloudy amber coloured liquid from a large polythene container, which was hidden away in a cupboard. 'See what you think to this. I brewed it myself.'

He handed one glass to me and started to make for the armchair opposite.

'On second thoughts, I'd better not sit down here in these clothes. They're a bit oily. Would you mind waiting whilst I change? I shall only be a couple of minutes. I love working on my cars but I'm not sure that car mechanics and dentistry go together. I have terrible trouble keeping my hands looking clean.'

'Do you have several cars?' I asked, thinking that dentistry must be quite a lucrative profession to be able to own more than one car. At the moment I couldn't even think about buying one.

'I have five if you can call the half-built Morgan three-wheeler a car. In fact, it's little more than a chassis at present.'

I had heard of Morgan cars before and whilst I didn't know much about them I somehow had the impression they were quite desirable in their own way. I wasn't too sure about the three-wheeler bit though; it tended to conjure up images of a Reliant Robin. 'What are your other cars?'

'They are all vintage,' replied Spencer somewhat pompously. 'I've got two Rolls Royces, a Bentley, a Frazer Nash and the Morgan three-wheeler which I bought a couple of months ago.'

'Not an Alfa Romeo?' I inquired looking at his T-shirt.

'No, not an Alfa. One of my friends in the Vintage Sports Car Club gave me this shirt. I said it was probably the only thing Alfa Romeo ever produced that wouldn't go rusty.'

He picked up his glass and took a long drink. 'I'll be back very soon.' As I looked round the room, it was obvious that his love of vintage cars was very profound. There were black and white photographs of them on the walls and his bookshelves were full of books on the subject. There were model cars as ornaments, bits of pistons as ashtrays and motor magazines scattered all round. Even the small grey rug in front of the fireplace had a red and black vintage sports car on it.

When Spencer returned he was wearing a pale green shirt, a red cravat and what looked like newer versions of the same corduroy trousers and suede shoes. He was still puffing on his pipe.

'What do you think of the beer? Do you like it?'

'It's very good indeed,' I enthused, though I was no authority. Beer was beer as far as I was concerned; it all tasted much the same to me. 'Do you brew a lot?'

'Yes I do. I started when I was an impoverished student thinking that it would save me some money. Instead of that, I spent just as much and drank a hell of a lot more than I would have done if I'd been buying pub beer. I like to think that over the years I have become a bit of an expert on brewing and now I don't really like any other beer as much as my own.'

He picked up his glass and sat in the armchair opposite.

'Do you have a car?'

'I'm afraid not. I can't afford one at the moment,' I replied.

'Don't worry, you soon will. I didn't have a car when I was a student, though I did have an old motorbike. It wasn't very reliable; the engine was in bits more than it was on the bike. I used to work on it in the kitchen of the house I shared with four other students. None of us was very tidy; in fact, the place was an absolute tip most of the time. The landlord was completely fed up with us and decided to try and sell the house. One day he came round with a prospective buyer, but he hadn't picked a good day and the house was even more of a shambles than usual; it was just like a pigsty. In sheer desperation he tried to impress the buyer by directing his attention to the cooker, which was relatively new. The landlord knew damn well that we never did any cooking so he thought that at least this might look presentable. He opened the oven door to reveal the cylinder head of my bike which I had placed in the oven to dry off after degreasing it and washing it down.'

'Don't you have a modern car at all, then?' I asked, thinking that vintage cars weren't very practical for everyday use.

'No, I'm not the slightest bit interested in modern cars; I wouldn't have one if you gave it to me. I like to buy old wrecks and rebuild them. This is what the Morgan was like when I bought it.' He handed me a photograph of what looked like a heap of scrap metal. 'Before you go, I'll show you what it's like now.'

'How many cars have you rebuilt?'

'Three. This will be my fourth. To be absolutely honest, the first two – my Bentley and the one I call my little Rolls – I didn't rebuild completely. They weren't in too bad a condition when I bought them; I just made them roadworthy. I did a fairly comprehensive rebuild job on my Frazer-Nash, though. That was in a pretty poor state when I got it. I'm also working on the big Rolls, which is going to need a lot of work on it before it's finished. It used to be a hearse but I've stripped off the body completely and I am going to rebuild it to look like a tourer of the same vintage. There was a fantastic oak platform that the coffin sat on. I wanted to make a coffee table out of it but Daphne, that's my wife, refused to have it in the house. I can't imagine why. Oak is oak. I can't see that it matters what it was used for previously, but I couldn't change her mind.

'Anyway, I'd better talk to you about the job and show you the surgeries. The practice was started by my father in 1946, in the good old days before the National Health Service. He ran it single-handed until I joined him, nearly ten years ago, in 1963. He retired four months ago. I can't cope with his patients as well as my own so I am looking for an associate to help me out. There is plenty of work here; the new associate will be fairly fully-committed, though he will probably be able to find room to take on new patients of his own, as well as father's old ones. I do quite a lot of private work as well as National Health, and as far as I'm concerned, you or whoever comes here, will have complete clinical freedom to treat patients as they see fit. Come and look at the surgeries.'

He led the way upstairs.

'Both surgeries are upstairs which can be a bit of a problem as we have a lot of elderly patients, but we usually manage one way or another. Most of the old ones are for dentures anyway, so you can treat them downstairs in the sitting room, if necessary. This is my surgery.'

He opened the first door at the top of the stairs revealing a light and spacious room painted in the same dove grey paint as the entrance hall. To the left of the door was a writing desk scattered with patients' record cards, National Health Service forms and other papers. In front of the main window, and facing it, was the most antiquated dental chair I had ever seen. It was rather like a barber's chair with shining black leather upholstery but it looked back-breakingly upright compared with the reclining couch-like chairs I had been used to at the dental hospital. It was not electrically controlled like most dental chairs; this one was operated by compressed air. To the left of it was a stout grey pedestal bearing a vitreous spittoon bowl and sprouting from the pedestal, like branches of a Christmas tree, were a bracket table, an operating light, and an old cord-driven drill unit which appeared to hang menacingly over the chair like an instrument of torture. To my great surprise, it struck a note of fear and my stomach turned over. I wondered if it had the same effect on the patients. Hopefully not, as it appeared that most of them had been patients of the practice for many years and didn't know any different. But to me, it was a stark reminder of the days when dentistry was a painful and extremely unpleasant experience. I felt as if I had stepped back in time. It was certainly very different from the equipment I had been trained on, and appeared positively ancient by comparison.

I was sure that I had seen a surgery just like it somewhere before. Was it like the ones I used to visit when I went for dental treatment as a child? No it wasn't; it was older even than that. It finally came to me; there was a very similar set-up in the Victoria and Albert Museum.

'I suppose the equipment looks a bit dated compared with what you are used to,' said Spencer, who seemed to have read my thoughts. 'It was all bought by my father in 1946. It's what he used throughout the whole of his career and is as good today as the day it was installed. It very rarely gives any trouble, which is very important in general practice. If your equipment lets you down you can't work and if you don't work you don't earn any money. I wouldn't give tuppence for a modern unit; they just aren't reliable. But this is so solidly made I'm convinced it will go on forever.

'This surgery is at the front of the house which is very useful because I can see what cars the patients are driving when they arrive.' With a twinkle in his eye he added, 'the type of car gives a good indication of their financial status and I adjust my fee scale accordingly.

'The other surgery, which is the one you would use if you come here to work, is at the side of the house but it has a very pleasant outlook; it gets the sun in the afternoon. The equipment in there isn't quite as old as this and I've made one or two modifications to it because I realise that someone fresh from university will probably be used to something a bit more up-to date.'

I noted that he did not say that he had bought any new equipment, and I had a strong feeling that it was going to be just as antiquated. I was, however, prepared to suspend judgement until after I'd seen it. He led me out of his surgery, turned left along the passageway and opened a door to reveal another room painted in the same shade of grey.

The room was somewhat smaller but still a good size with a large window overlooking the drive and the garden of the house next door. The seat of the dental chair had been converted so that the patient could lie down which was the way I had been used to working. Some of the other items of equipment had been re-sited so that they would reach the new position, though it seemed to me at first sight that the degree of reorganisation was probably not sufficient to cater for all eventualities, but without actually using the surgery it was impossible to foresee all the possible difficulties. The general feel of the surgery was very much the same as Spencer's and the most striking feature was an old cord-driven drill which, until now, I had considered to be virtually obsolete.

As tactfully as I could, I raised the question, 'Do you not think that the modern electric or air motors, which don't have all these arms and pulleys and are much less conspicuous to the patients, are a lot less frightening?'

Spencer brushed the suggestion aside. 'It doesn't seem to worry them. In any case, the modern drills are much too flimsy for my liking. This one will go on forever and needs practically no maintenance. Last week I used it to drill some steel brackets for my Morgan. You wouldn't be able to do that with a modern drill; it would never stand up to it.'

As he was speaking my attention was drawn to the electric power socket in the corner of the room by the window. Spencer noticed I was looking at it.

'Unfortunately there is only one power point in this room so everything has to come from it,' he explained.

There were adapters within adapters within adapters; in all, about eight plugs leading wires in all directions. The complete assembly stuck out from the wall by a good six inches and I was particularly intrigued by one thick wire, which ran upwards to the window and to the outside through a hole in the frame.

'That one feeds power to my workshop and garage,' said Spencer. 'I must admit that it's not an ideal arrangement but as long as you don't switch everything on at the same time it's unlikely that you'll overload the circuit. Most of the things plugged in here don't take much current. I keep saying that I'll get the electrics in this house sorted out; more power points installed. In fact the whole place probably needs rewiring. It's just getting around to doing it. There are lots of other things which need doing like having central heating installed, but to be honest, my cars are much more important, so everything else tends to take a back seat.'

'What do you do for heating now?' I asked, thinking that it was a big house and must be cold in winter. I was also very concerned about how the outdated electrical system would cope with the widespread use of electric heaters. 'It has to be warm for the patients.'

'Oh it's warm enough. Most patients are in a bit of a sweat anyway at the prospect of coming here. There are gas fires in the surgeries and waiting room. For the rest of the house we rely on the heat generated by light bulbs,' he replied with a wry smile.

I was beginning to enjoy his dry sense of humour. He came across as being friendly, good-natured and in spite of all the shortcomings of the surgery equipment, I was already beginning to think that working with him would probably be good fun. He obviously didn't seem to take life too seriously and whilst there is no doubt that dentistry can be a stressful job there was very little sign that he was unduly stressed by it. I must admit that I wasn't looking to join a high-powered sort of practice; I wanted to be able to work at a fairly leisurely pace carrying out the sort of dentistry I had been trained to do.

'I suppose you work sitting down?' he asked, in a tone which suggested that he thought it was a ridiculous way to operate.

'Yes, I do. That's the way we're taught these days.'

'I thought you probably would though I have never really been able to adapt to that way of working myself. In any case, patients hate lying down for their treatment; they would much rather sit upright. All dentists worked standing up when I did my training and I still do most of the time, but I thought that if I employed someone newly qualified they would want to sit down to it, so, with this in mind, I installed a swivelling stool. I designed it myself and I must say that I am rather proud of it. One of its great advantages is that there is such a good height adjustment on it you can have the patient either sitting up or lying down. I've actually got one in my surgery now. I don't use it all the time yet but I find I am using it more and more. Try it and see what you think.'

I had never seen anything quite like it before. The stools I had been used to had castors, which enabled you to move around freely, but Spencer had dreamed up a completely different system. There was a small round stool with a platform for the feet and the whole thing was fixed to a pivoting arm, which swung around behind the dental chair. The stool was quite high off the floor and I had to stretch to reach it. As I tried to mount it I put too much pressure on the side of the stool which immediately swung away from me at a terrifying speed, causing me to deposit my entire weight suddenly, unexpectedly and extremely painfully on the surgery floor.

'You have to be careful getting on and off because it pivots very freely,' advised Spencer who was obviously more concerned with promoting his invention than with my welfare.

'Yes it does, doesn't it,' I agreed, feeling more than a little ruffled by the experience.

'Try again,' he urged, 'it's fine once you get used to it.'

This time I stabilised myself by clinging tightly to the dental chair as I mounted the stool. Taking great care to position myself centrally over it, I slowly lowered myself down. Warily and extremely unsteadily, I let go of the chair and there I was, perched at what seemed like a fantastic height above the floor looking down on everything around me. The slightest movement or a mere shift of weight caused the stool to swing alarmingly.

'I feel a bit unstable,' I exclaimed wondering how one could possibly carry out dentistry balanced precariously up there.

'It takes a little while to get used to it but it's great after a bit of practice. It's like riding a bike; once you have mastered it you'll think it's easy. You'll see that there's room on the foot platform for the pedal unit for the drills, so you don't have to stretch down to the floor. Everything is up there with you and you can swing almost a hundred and eighty degrees right around the back of the chair. Don't you think it's a brilliant idea?'

'Er, yes, it's an excellent idea,' I replied dubiously, 'once you get used to it.'

I was about to discover that getting off was just as hazardous as getting on because I had not realised, and Spencer had not told me, that that the pivot arm was fitted with a powerful spring to return it to the central position. As I alighted, the stool swung swiftly away from me and then, under the power of the spring, returned even more rapidly. The edge of the substantial metal platform smartly rapped my right ankle, causing me to cry out in pain.

'I'm sorry,' Spencer apologised, looking genuinely concerned this time. 'I should have warned you about that. Anyway, you know how to operate it now. You will find that it makes life very much easier once you've got used to using it. How does this equipment compare with what you had at university?'

'Well,' I began, searching for the right words so as not to hurt his feelings, but hoping that I could give a reasonably truthful answer. 'It is rather older than the equipment at the dental hospital. The Dean was always most anxious that we should have the very latest equipment, but a lot of it was badly made and not at all reliable.'

'Exactly,' responded Spencer, 'that is why I am hanging on to all this. Take my X-ray machine for example. Come and look at this.'

He led me into another large room, which overlooked the back garden. 'This is the office and X-ray room. We keep patients' record cards in here,' pointing to the filing cabinets. 'And here is the X-ray machine. Father bought it just after the war. They don't make them like this anymore.'

'They certainly don't,' I reiterated, gazing in awe at its sheer magnitude. I had never seen anything like it before; it was many times bigger than the X-ray machines I had been used to at the hospital. I now realised why it was in a separate room. It was so colossal, it could not possibly have fitted into a surgery. Although the room in which it was situated was quite big, it looked extremely crowded as it contained two small desks, the filing cabinets for the patients' records and an old dental chair for the patient being X-rayed to sit in. The chair was completely dwarfed by the huge, gleaming black monster.

'It will go on forever,' exclaimed Spencer. 'Just look at the size of the head and feel the weight of it. The modern ones are only a fraction of the size. This machine is so solidly made, it really is a fantastic piece of engineering.'

'How do you set the exposure time?' I inquired looking somewhat sceptically at the primitive control panel. The machines I had been used to all had timers calibrated in fractions of a second so that the exposure time could be varied according to the part of the mouth being X-rayed. This was necessary in order to obtain a properly exposed radiograph.

'Oh you don't need to worry about adjusting the exposure time with this machine like you do with the modern ones, you just press the button and I'll guarantee you will get a perfectly exposed X-ray every time. It doesn't matter whether it's a back tooth, front tooth or whatever.'

'Really? That's amazing.' I replied, trying not to appear too incredulous. There was one thing on which I could agree, however; 'It certainly looks very strongly made.'

'Most definitely,' said Spencer. 'Reliable equipment – that's what you need in general practice. There is nothing more infuriating than things which keep breaking down and, as I said before, if the equipment lets you down, you can't work, and that costs you money.

'Anyway, now that you've seen the surgeries let's go back downstairs and have another beer, and you can tell me how you feel about coming here to work.'

He ushered me back to the sitting room still blowing out great clouds of smoke. He poured out two more beers and we sat down.

'I was thinking of paying an associate forty five percent of gross income. How does that sound to you? Is that the sort of percentage other principals are offering?'

'Well,' I began, hesitating slightly at first but then thinking that as I was not yet convinced whether or not I wanted the job, I might as well drive as hard a bargain as possible. 'I understand from many of my friends that many associates are getting fifty percent'

'Are they really?' Spencer replied without much surprise in his voice. ' Okay. Fifty percent it is, then . The job is yours if you want it.'

I was completely taken aback by the suddenness of his decision. 'Just like that?'

'Why not? You seem all right to me, I feel sure that you will fit in very well here. In any case, I'm desperate. Ever since father retired, I have been absolutely rushed off my feet. I can't carry on much longer without some help. Do you want the job?'

I didn't really know what to say. 'Surely you will want references before taking me on? Can I think about it overnight and let you know tomorrow?'

'Of course you can . Give me a ring about lunchtime. As far as the references are concerned, I'll contact your Dean, but I'm sure he'll write about you in glowing terms. I think I'm a pretty good judge of character and I'm quite satisfied with what I've seen. Where are you staying tonight?'

'I'm booked in at the King's Arms Hotel.'

'You should be comfortable there . It's quite a nice hotel. Enjoy your stay.'

He showed me to the door. 'I hope you decide to come and join me, I think we'll get on well together.'

'Thanks for the beers and for showing me round. I promise I'll phone about one-thirty tomorrow with my decision. Good-bye.' We shook hands and I left.

CHAPTER THREE

I had been having such difficulty in making up my mind . Would I possibly be able to decide by tomorrow? I thought about the ancient equipment and the stupid operating stool, the antiquated X-ray machine which looked as if it wasn't even safe to use. Was this really what I wanted? I wasn't at all convinced. I did, however, like Spencer and he would pay me well, which was something I had to consider in view of my financial situation. I felt sure that life would be a lot of fun with him around. I got the impression that his approach to dentistry was simple, down-to earth and matter-of-fact, and I had a strong suspicion that his methods would be just as outdated as his equipment, though I was only guessing about that. His practice was certainly not the place to be if one wanted to be at the forefront of technology or had ambitions to make a name for oneself in the world of general practice dentistry, but I have to say that I found his attitude quite refreshing and, in a strange sort of way, very appealing. Many of the academics I had been in contact with over the past few years were, in fact, very narrow people who had no interests whatsoever outside dentistry. Spencer was a more complete person who obviously enjoyed life and was able to keep things in perspective Dentistry was just a part of this life, not the whole of it.

Dentistry can be a very stressful job. Apparently the suicide rate amongst dentists is very high and many of them experience drink and drug problems. It seemed most unlikely that Spencer would fall victim to any of this – not with his philosophy on life. His practice was a complete contrast to everything the hospital stood for and with which I had been indoctrinated for the past six years. I had been wondering whether I was ready for a change and working for Spencer would not just be a change – it would be like going into another world.

By the time I had reached the hotel I had made up my mind and I decided to phone him straight away.

'I don't need until tomorrow. I have decided I would like to come and work for you.'

'That's great,' he replied at the other end of the phone. 'Why don't you pop back after dinner this evening and we can sort out a few details?'

'Yes, I'd like to. I'll see you later.'

'Good. You can also have a look at my cars whilst you're here. I didn't have time to show them to you this afternoon.'

I put down the phone and the feeling that a great weight had been lifted from me suddenly came over me. I had made the decision, and, whilst there were sure to be some reservations, I felt deep down inside that I had done the right thing. I lay on my bed for a while feeling quite excited about the future.

The hotel was, as Spencer had predicted, most comfortable, with a homely and informal atmosphere. It suited my requirements perfectly. I had a relaxing bath before enjoying an excellent meal in the spacious dining room to the muted accompaniment of Bach's Concertos for harpsichord and strings.

When I arrived back at Spencer's house at about 8.30 p.m. his wife answered the door.

'Hello, you must be Justin,' she said pleasantly. 'Do come in. I'm Daphne. Spencer is where you will usually find him at this time in the evening; in his workshop, working on his cars. Come in and sit down and I'll give him a call.'

She invited me into the kitchen and hailed Spencer on an intercom arrangement, which was connected to his workshop.

'Send him down here,' I heard Spencer say.

The workshop was an extension to the garage, which was built at the side of the house. When I got there, Spencer was lying on his back underneath the chassis of a huge Rolls Royce.

'You came just at the right time,' he called out. 'I need the assistance of an extra pair of strong hands at this very moment. I am hoping that you will use the strength that you have developed by extracting teeth to help me extract the gearbox from this car.'

A few moments later I was lying alongside him, heaving and straining, and just as covered in oil as he was.

'It's so much easier with someone to help,' he panted. 'It would have taken me at least two hours on my own . With your help, we'll have this gearbox on the bench in no time at all.'

Half an hour later, we were standing upright with aching arms and backs but satisfied to think that the mighty Rolls Royce gearbox had been delivered, with the help of some lifting equipment, safely on to the workbench.

'Thanks very much,' said Spencer, 'splendid effort. I told you we would have it out in no time. Oh, by the way, I'm so delighted that you've decided to come and join the practice.'

'I hope it turns out well for both of us,' I replied. 'I thought it was going to be a difficult decision to make but something told me to go for it.'

'Well, I'm sure it was the right decision. I think we'll get along together just fine, especially now that I know you're a bit of a dab hand at removing gearboxes.'

He suddenly became aware of the oily state of my hands, face and clothes. 'You had better come into the house and clean up. My patients are used to me being a bit oily, but it wouldn't do for you to begin your career in general practice looking more like a motor mechanic than a dentist. The people in this area can be very demanding and until they get used to you, you will be under very close scrutiny.'

The words 'under very close scrutiny' struck a slight note of fear in my heart. I was very much aware that although I had passed the necessary examinations to be able to say that I was qualified to practise dentistry, at the same time I was very lacking in experience and it would take some time to build up my confidence. Going out into general practice would be like being thrown into the deep end of a swimming pool immediately after learning to swim. Spencer would have been in that situation himself a few years ago. I wondered if he remembered how it felt. I decided, however, not to ask him about it, as I didn't want him to think that I wasn't up to the job.

'Before we go in, I must show you my cars,' said Spencer with great enthusiasm. 'This is my little Rolls.'

In front of the huge Rolls Royce we had been working on and nearest to the garage entrance was a gleaming black and green Rolls Royce, which although much smaller was still quite a large vehicle.

'This is the car I use on a daily basis for going to the shops and the local pub.'

'It's beautiful, Spencer.' I ran my eyes over the immaculate paintwork, which had a depth of shine only seen on cars of a certain age. Then I noticed the tax disc. Before I could think whether it was polite to mention it I blurted out, 'but the tax disc is two years out of date.'

'I know it is,' he replied. 'I can't tax it because there is a problem with the suspension and until I get that sorted out I can't get an MOT. Without an MOT I can't get the road tax. I'll get it sorted eventually, but with a car like this you can get away with it. A policeman stopped me last week and I thought he was going to do me for having no tax but he stopped me because he was interested in the car and wanted to know how long I'd had it and where I got it from. He never mentioned the tax.'

'You were lucky.'

'Well, possibly, but as I said, with a car like this, tax is a minor consideration. Now here is my Frazer Nash. What do you think of this?'

Although it was obviously designed as a sports car, its outdated lines and general sit-up-and-beg appearance suggested that it wouldn't be all that fast by present day standards, there was nevertheless a certain amount of style about it.

'It looks great,' I replied. 'Do you use it much?'

'I do in the summer. I went to the French Alps in it last year and it ran like a dream. I'm hoping to take it to France again next spring.'

'There isn't much room for luggage.'

'You'd be surprised how much you can pack into it. You just have to make full use of all the available space. I always travel light, anyway. In any case, it's a good thing that Daphne is limited on how much she can take with her. She'd take the kitchen sink if she could.'

At the side of the Frazer Nash was a diminutive chassis. A great deal of work was obviously needed on it before it could be put on the road, but I could see that it was the skeleton of a small three-wheeled vehicle.

'This is my Morgan. It still needs a lot of work but I am really looking forward to driving it. I think it will be a lot of fun.'

I looked at the tiny cockpit and then at Spencer's slightly rotund figure, and couldn't help thinking that if he put on much more weight he would have great difficulty getting into the driving seat.

'Will it be very fast?'

'Well, not really by present day standards, but it will feel fast. Anyway let's go in so that you can clean up, and then we'll have a drink.'

He showed me the downstairs cloakroom where I washed the oil and grease off my hands as best I could, though it didn't come off easily. Afterwards I joined him and Daphne in their sitting room where I was presented with more of Spencer's home-brewed beer. We sat and chatted until well after midnight and I felt very relaxed and comfortable in their presence. After an hour or so, it was as if I had known them for years and as the evening wore on I felt increasingly certain that I had made the right decision by agreeing to come and work for Spencer.

They were extremely open about their lives and related to me how Spencer's father had bought the house because of its size and its position in order to establish a dental practice. Spencer and his brother had been born and brought up there and Spencer's parents lived in it until a couple of years ago when, in anticipation of Spencer's father's retirement, they had a house built at the bottom of the garden. Spencer's parents moved into the new house and Spencer bought the house containing the practice from his father at a very low price and at a very reasonable rate of interest. Spencer readily admitted that he had been very fortunate to come into possession of his own dental practice in this way and appreciated the fact that, because his financial commitments were low, he did not need to work desperately hard in order to pay his way. Most dentists of his age who owned their own practices would be much more heavily committed financially. That is not to say, however, that Spencer was not keen to earn money. I learnt that he had an expensive lifestyle, that he and Daphne loved entertaining, dining out and taking holidays, not to mention the money he spent on his cars.

I also learnt something about Spencer's little idiosyncrasies, such as the fact that every day after lunch he would go to bed for an hour. He had done this for years and it didn't matter whether he was at work or away on holiday – he always had an hour's sleep before beginning the afternoon. He wasn't content with sleeping in a chair; he actually undressed and got into bed. He claimed that it enabled him to stay up much later at night, which then gave him time to work longer on his cars. It was clear that Daphne found the habit a little bit irritating, especially when they were on holiday or were going out somewhere together.

'I feel like throwing a bucket of water over him sometimes,' she said jokingly, though I could see that there was more than a hint of truth in what she was saying. 'He has always had a sleep after lunch as long as I've known him and I don't think I'm ever going to change him now.'

'Our sleeping patterns seem to be totally incompatible,' Spencer interjected rather seriously. 'Daphne gave up her job as a secretary two years ago and now takes on typing work at home, but instead of working during the day like most people, she starts work at about ten o'clock in the evening and works through until two or three in the morning.'

'Well that means I can do other things during the day like shopping for your food, dear,' quipped Daphne.

'That is true,' Spencer conceded, 'but as you don't normally get up until midday, you don't get much done in the mornings.'

There was a slight edge to Spencer's voice as he said it, but Daphne merely defended her position without attempting to retaliate.

'One of the advantages of doing freelance work is that you can work whichever hours you want. I seem to be able to work most efficiently late at night, but I do also need a certain amount of sleep.'

'I suppose I get a bit envious when I have to get up to work in the surgery on a cold winter's morning and you just roll over and go back to sleep,' said Spencer wistfully.

'At least you don't have to travel anywhere. I've seen him get up at five to nine when his first patient is at nine o'clock and already in the waiting room. Some dentists have to travel miles to their practices. It's lucky that Beryl is so reliable; that's Spencer's nurse. She's always here well before nine o'clock and is able to let the patients in if Spencer hasn't surfaced.'

There was no apparent animosity between them, and I got the impression that each one accepted the other's little quirks, though not without some slight irritation at times. We had been so engrossed in conversation that I hadn't realised how time had passed until I glanced at the clock above the stone fireplace.

'My goodness, is that the time? I'm sorry I've stayed so long. Have I kept you from your work, Daphne?'

'No, not at all, Justin. As I said, when you are freelance you can work whenever you want to. I might just do an hour or so before I go to bed but I don't intend it to be a long session; there is no desperate hurry for the work I have on hand at the moment. It can wait until tomorrow.'

'Well, I must be going anyway. I'm setting off back home tomorrow quite early.'

They saw me to the door and I stepped out into the darkness of the village. Few places were lit up now and in the absence of streetlights it was very difficult to see much at all. I realised that when I moved to Luccombury I would have to get into the habit of carrying a torch around with me.

CHAPTER FOUR

I was awakened by the metallic clunk of my letterbox and as soon as I heard the dull sickening thud of the envelope landing on the floor, I knew instinctively that it was a letter from my bank manager. I'm not sure exactly how I knew, but somehow his letters seemed to produce a distinctive and unpleasant sound. Unfortunately, it was a sound that had become very familiar to me over the past few weeks. I did not really need to open the envelope; I was well aware that it would bring bad news and would most likely demand that I make an immediate appointment to see him to discuss my ever-worsening financial situation. I knew that the most upsetting thing about it would be that it would undoubtedly contain sordid details of the exact depth of the abyss into which my impecuniosity had plummeted.

My speculations were alarmingly accurate and the tone of the letter left me in no doubt that I must respond without delay. I was so unsettled that I felt it necessary to phone the bank even before I sat down to my coffee and cereal. I discovered that the manager was every bit as anxious to see me as I had feared, and the degree of urgency demanded that I make an appointment for that very morning. I had already had some fairly unpleasant meetings with the bank manager and, as I am the sort of person who dislikes any sort of confrontation, I regret to say that the prospect of seeing him ruined my breakfast.

'Sit down, Mr Derwent.'

His manner was even more sombre than the last time I saw him and was, I felt, on the verge of being threatening.

'I really cannot allow you to continue overdrawing on your account as you are doing at present. I know that you have been a student for a long time and that it has not been easy for you but you must appreciate that the bank needs some sort of security before it can allow borrowing to this extent. I regret to have to say that I think the time has come to freeze all spending at the present time and it will be necessary for you to arrange for someone to act as guarantor for your overdraft before I can consider increasing it any further.'

'Well, Mr Palfry, I am very sorry that my overdraft has increased so dramatically, but it has honestly been due to essential expenditure. Hopefully, however, the situation will improve very shortly now that I am qualified and will soon be starting work.'

He did not appear to be particularly excited by the news.

'I offer you my congratulations on passing your finals, Mr Derwent. I am delighted to hear that you have been successful.'

He spoke without a trace of emotion.

'However, the last time you were here you intimated that you would probably be staying on at the hospital and taking a job as a house surgeon. I have to say that I was somewhat disappointed to hear that this was your intention. I do not think that you will find an academic career at all lucrative and, certainly in the early days, it will be far from it. In fact, it will be some considerable time before you start to earn anything like a reasonable income and, for this reason, the bank must look at your financial situation with a good deal of caution. To put it bluntly, your decision to take a post as house surgeon at the hospital, in my opinion, renders your financial prospects fairly unpromising in the short term at least. Unfortunately, you have already incurred debts which are substantial enough to cause the bank to be more than a little anxious as to how you are going to clear them. Your decision to stay on at the hospital does nothing to allay this anxiety. As I said, the bank will need to protect its investment in you and, for this reason, it will be necessary for you to provide a guarantor before you can increase your overdraft beyond its present level and we shall also be expecting to see a steady but definite reduction in your level of borrowing over the next few months.'

'I've decided not to stay on at the hospital. I have taken a job in general practice.'

It took a few moments for my words to sink in, and then quite suddenly his demeanour changed. It was a dramatic and radical transformation.

'Well, Mr Derwent, this throws a very different light upon everything. I am absolutely certain that you have made a very wise decision. I feel sure, though it was not my place to say so, that general practice is a much more sensible path for you to take. It will undoubtedly bring you financial security at a very early stage of your career, and – let's not beat about the bush, Mr Derwent – financial security in these difficult times is a very valuable commodity. I am delighted that you have seen sense and put all ideas of a hospital career behind you. I am sure you will never look back, and there are lots of ways in which the bank will be able to assist you to manage your affairs. I look forward to a long and fruitful relationship.'

He pressed the button on his intercom and spoke to his secretary. 'Miss Blake, will you send in coffee and biscuits for two please? Now tell me, Mr Derwent, where are you going to be working?'

'In Luccombury, in Dorset.'

'Really? How lovely. I know it well. I lived quite near there for several years. It's a beautiful part of the country. I'm sure you will be extremely happy. I loved the quaint little old stone cottages and the wonderful views from the town square of green fields and trees, which completely surround the town. I'm quite envious of you. I must admit that I would prefer to be a bank manager somewhere like that instead of in this huge city, but we can't always have what we want and I must not complain.'

In all the years I had been dealing with the bank I had never seen him in such an amiable mood. The news about my move into general practice obviously resulted in him seeing my financial situation from an entirely fresh viewpoint.

'Oh yes, this throws an entirely different light on the way the bank views your financial prospects. In the circumstances, I think it will be quite in order to double your present overdraft facility and if you find that this is not sufficient to meet your needs just let me know and we can discuss it further. I am sure we will be able to come to some agreement.'

'Will I still need a guarantor?' I asked thinking that it would not be at all easy to find someone I could ask to take on this role for me.

'No, no. That won't be necessary in the circumstances. You are, however, going to need a cheque guarantee card, which I will arrange to have sent to you within the next day or so. This will allow you much freer use of your current account. I think also that you will probably find a credit card useful, but be careful how you use it as it's very easy to get carried away and overspend. I am sure, however, that I can rely on you to use it sensibly. If you fill in this form now, I will see that it is processed as quickly as possible and the card sent to you without delay.'

I drank my coffee with Mr Palfry and chatted to him in a way that we had never chatted before. Many people had said to me that being a dental surgeon carried with it a certain status and for the first time, I was beginning to understand what they meant. I was made to feel that I was now a customer of some importance to the bank. They actually wanted me to continue to bank with them. Previously, I had been made to feel that they were definitely doing me a favour by keeping my account and that I had to comply strictly with all their constraints. Although I had exactly the same amount of money, albeit a negative amount, when I left the bank that morning as when I entered it three quarters of an hour previously, I suddenly felt infinitely more affluent and my former financial worries had magically dissolved during that memorable interview with Mr Palfry.

For the past six years I had been able to spend money only on essentials, I had not allowed myself to think about buying anything, which could even remotely be considered a luxury item. Suddenly, I found myself wondering how best to make use of my newfound wealth. I would need to find somewhere to live, but now my financial circumstances would allow me to look for somewhere nice instead of having to accept the cheapest accommodation available. It crossed my mind that I might even be able to buy a car. It wouldn't be the most sensible thing to do - even an old one would swallow up most of the agreed overdraft figure – but I did want a car so badly. Perhaps I could get one on hire purchase. It was not long before I had convinced myself that car ownership, one way or another, was a distinct possibility.

I walked back to the university common room, which was now unusually quiet. I realised that most students, including my friends, had gone home to visit their families and life was becoming a bit lonely around the university. It reinforced my feelings that my time there had finally run out and that I should make the break and move on, so I decided to travel down to Luccombury and spend a few days there before actually starting work. I needed to find somewhere to live and it would be nice to have time to feel my way around the area.

CHAPTER FIVE

When I arrived back in Luccombury for the second time in the space of a fortnight, I noticed that there had been a marked change in temperature. There was now a distinct nip in the air and, although the weather was still bright, the weak November sun was without much warmth and the days were becoming depressingly short.

Spencer and Daphne had been kind enough to let me stay with them and I spent a very pleasant time wandering around the town and surrounding area, soaking up the country atmosphere. I soon realised that I was becoming very fond of Luccombury. It was a unique town with a long history, almost totally encircled by hills and situated in the most beautiful part of Dorset. So far it had been completely untouched by the destructive hands of developers and only the television aerials and cars parked in the square served as a reminder that this was the 1970s.

My half-hearted attempts to find permanent accommodation had not been successful after three days and just when I was beginning to think that the situation was becoming serious, Spencer came to the rescue.

'Go and see this chap. I don't know him personally but I've heard through a patient that he has a cottage to let. It might be just what you are looking for. His name is Ephraim Trivett and he lives down a wooded track on the outskirts of the town.'

'That's an unusual name,' I remarked.

'It's a good old country name and I rather gather that he is something of a country character. Anyway, it might be worth your while paying him a visit.'

I decided that it was good advice and later that day I set off to look for his house. I found it without too much difficulty though it was a bit off the beaten track. He lived in a delightful little stone cottage with a thatched roof surrounded by trees and open fields. There were two other similar cottages alongside and the group of them formed a small community just at the edge of the main town, though their position was such that it appeared that they were miles from any other civilisation.

As I approached, a flock of racing pigeons circled the sky above me and finally landed on the roof of a shed at the bottom of the garden to the cottage. A short, slim figure emerged from the shed and greeted me. It appeared that he was expecting me.

He was a typical countryman; unshaven, with small black-rimmed spectacles, wearing a cloth cap, thick checked shirt and a tattered old sweater. I got the impression that washing did not rate too highly on his list of priorities. He was probably in his early forties but looked quite a bit older, due mainly to his sun-dried and weather-beaten complexion. When he opened his mouth my first thought was that if everyone living in the area felt the same way about dentists as he obviously did, then it was not going to be easy to make a living. It was clear that he had never sought dental treatment because all he had was a row of black stumps broken off at gum level.

''Ee come to see cottage?'

'That's right, if it's not inconvenient.'

'Noah, not a bit. 'Tis 'long here. Come on, I'll show 'ee round.'

The cottage he was letting was about fifty yards further up the track, hidden from Ephraim's and the other two cottages by a cluster of trees. It was semi-detached and an absolute dream. It was appropriately called 'Ivy Cottage' as the three hundred year old bulging stone walls were completely covered with ivy. It had a beautiful old oak door, which opened directly into a spacious living room with a flagstone floor, beamed ceiling and an enormous inglenook fireplace. In the corner of the room, winding up behind the fireplace, a rickety staircase led upstairs to two small bedrooms and a bathroom.

''Twas put on mains drainage last year,' announced Ephraim proudly, 'an' there's room to park yer car o'er yon.'

'I don't have a car at the moment but I am hoping to get one soon.' I replied wistfully.

'Only 'ad mine a week. Wrote my last one off on bend out by Moorgate Farm. Do 'ee know it?'

'No, not really. I'm new to the area.'

'Helluva blind bend. Mind 'ee, I were doing 'bout sixty in middle of road, like, and chap comin' other way weren't 'xactly crawlin' neither. Wrote 'is car off an' all. People are allus havin' smashes on narrer roads round 'ere; can't be avoided.'

'Whose fault was it? It sounds as though it might have been yours.'

'Probably were, but 'tis never worth arguin' about. Tends to work on knock-for-knock basis round 'ere, see?'

'Knock-for-knock?' I exclaimed.

'Yeah, knock-for-knock. It means 'ee pays for own damage, like.'

'I know what it means, I just don't like the sound of it. It doesn't exactly encourage careful driving, does it?'

'There bain't much careful drivin' round 'ere. People are in too much of hurry, see?'

'I thought life in the country was supposed to be leisurely.'

'Well 'tis, but not on th'road. Could be that folk want a bit of excitement, like, when they drive. I know I does. I allus say 'tis never worth 'avin' a good car, 'tis best to have an old banger, then don't matter what happens to it. I paid twenty quid for mine. I can drive it as fast and as recklessly as I likes and don't need worry about it. I'll give 'ee the name of the chap I bought it from if 'ee wants it. Specialises in buyin' up old wrecks and puttin' 'em back on th'road. He's real cheap, like.'

I had rather hoped that my first car might be something rather more decent, but I was filled with horror at the prospect of taking out my pride and joy and meeting someone like Ephraim, driving like a maniac on one of the many narrow bends in the area.

'What does 'ee do for a livin'?' Ephraim asked. 'Don't look as though 'ee be used to gettin' yer hands dirty.'

'I'm a dentist,' I replied, thinking that the title of 'dental surgeon' might sound a bit too ostentatious. 'I've just qualified and I'm coming to work in Luccombury with Spencer Padginton.'

'Dentist? Good grief. There ain't much call for 'em round 'ere; nobody goes nowhere near. I don't believe in 'em, like. Our mother took I to have a tooth out when I were about ten. He pulled an' tugged at it but couldn't shift bugger; finally there were an almighty crack and damn thing broke into hundred pieces. That were enough for I, there were no way I were stayin' for any more o' that so I upped and left. By God, I were in agony for two weeks. I can still remember it as if 'twere yesterday, like. I vowed then that I would never go near a dentist ever again and never have. Rest o' tooth he broke is still 'ere and I lost all these when I came off a motorbike.'

He lifted his lip to display a revolting row of rotting black roots. 'I were drunk at time like so didn't feel a thing. This were on the bend by Synderford Farm one night after I'd drunk 'bout nine pints o' scrumpy and a few whiskies in Three Horseshoes. A car were comin' in opposite direction, like and as the road weren't wide enough for both o' us, I had to swerve to avoid him, see? Can't remember much else 'bout it.

'He obviously didn't hit I or 'twould have been curtains, like, but I was lyin' in road unconscious till 'bout five o'clock next mornin'. When I came to, got up, dusted I down, then jumped on bike and rode home. First thing our mother said when she saw I was, 'what happened to yer teeth?' I looked in mirror and saw that I didn't 'ave none no more. Folk round here don't bother much with dentists. I shouldn't think 'ee'll get much work.'

As I stood talking to him I was aware that his car, which was parked nearby, was bouncing up and down. It took a few moments before I realised why and saw a black face staring out through the windscreen.

'Is that your dog in the car?' I asked. 'He doesn't seem very happy about being shut in.'

'She wants to be out 'ere, right enough like, but I has to be careful, see; she don't take to everyone. If she don't happen to like 'ee she'll just as soon take a lump out o' yer leg.'

For a brief moment I was slightly apprehensive as he opened the car door, but as soon as I saw her wagging tail, I knew that I had nothing to fear from her. She ran over to me and immediately began licking my hand.

'What's her name?' I asked stroking the wiry black fur on the stockily-built mongrel's head.

'Nellie. She's taken a real likin' to 'ee, which is just as well; she can be real mean when she wants to be. Her biggest hatred though is cats; can't stand 'em, see? If she spots one she'll be off after 'im like a rat up a drainpipe and there's not a thing I can do stop her. Killed next door's ginger tom. Tried to call her off but 'twere no good. She's a real terror. He weren't first cat she's killed, like. If 'ee come to live here, don't bring a cat with 'ee or she'll 'ave it.'

I looked into Nellie's soft brown eyes, and from the way she was nuzzling up to me and licking my hand, I found it very hard to believe that what Ephraim was telling me had any truth in it. Whatever she was like, there was no doubt that I certainly had nothing to fear from her.

'Any'ow, what does 'ee think to cottage: is 'ee interested in it?'

'Definitely, I think it is wonderful. How much is the rent?'

'Eight quid a week and rates on top.'

'I'll take it.'

'That's good. 'ere, 'ee 'ad just as well take key right now, 'ee might want to bring some furniture round, though folk round here don't bother much 'bout lockin' doors; 'ee ain't likely to get broken into.'

'I haven't actually got any furniture yet, but I can soon get some. When can I move in?'

''Ee's got key, 'ee can move in when 'ee likes; right 'way if 'ee wants to. I 'ave one or two pieces 'ee can put in there for the time bein' 'til 'ee gets sorted out. I'll stick in a table and couple o' chairs; 'ee probably won't need much more 'an that for a start, like, and I'll chop some logs for 'ee. There's no 'eating 'cept for open fire, see, and it's turnin' cold now. Look at the frost on they fields; it ain't lifted all day.'

Until that moment, I had not noticed that the cottage was icy cold inside but it was so attractive and I could picture a roaring fire in the inglenook fireplace. I felt sure that it would be very cosy when it was lived in once again. I felt very pleased about renting the cottage and gave Ephraim four weeks rent in advance, then I set off at a brisk pace to tell Spencer and Daphne the good news. As I was making my way through the narrow winding streets I became even more aware of the fact that it was getting bitterly cold. I turned up the collar of my jacket and thrust my hands into my pockets. I was not really prepared for this sudden decrease in temperature and I wished I had brought a thicker coat with me. I suppose I had imagined that the weather in the south would be much warmer.

I reached the town centre where the frost-coated frames of the shop windows glistened in the frail amber glow from the lights outside the Red Lion Hotel. I quickened my pace, anxious to get back to warmth and comfort as quickly as possible but as I walked past a little electrical shop, a notice in the shop window caught my eye. It was advertising a special, once in a lifetime, never to be repeated offer, on a refrigerator.

Heaven knows why I suddenly became interested in buying a refrigerator. Obviously I would need one eventually but surely, there were other things more important than this that I needed to buy first. Nevertheless, I thought the fridge looked exceptionally well-made, about the right size, attractively styled and the price seemed so low, it was an offer too good to miss. After all, since there were so many things I would need to buy in the near future, I had to take full advantage of any special offers which came to my attention. Did it really matter what order I bought them in?

On an impulse, I went into the shop with only minutes to spare before it closed and promptly wrote out a cheque for the generously discounted purchase price of the appliance. I was quite disappointed when the shopkeeper said that he did not need to see my new cheque guarantee card.

'It's a genuine offer,' he claimed. 'These fridges have been specially imported from Russia; I am sure you will be very happy with it. The only problem is, I can't deliver it for you as I don't drive anymore. I can probably arrange transport for you if you can't carry it yourself but it might take a few days and there would have to be a charge.'

'Oh don't worry about that,' I proclaimed confidently. 'I don't have a car myself, but I'm sure I can find someone who will pick it up for me. Leave it to me, I'll arrange it as soon as I can.'

'Yes, all right, but bear in mind that it comes in quite a large box. I doubt if you would get it into an ordinary car. You'll need a van, really.'

I thanked him and reassured him once again that transport would not be a problem though I had no idea at the time how I was going to be able to get the fridge back to the cottage. I hurried off and arrived back at Fothergill House just in time for dinner.

Spencer was delighted to hear that the cottage had proved suitable and that I had been able to rent it, but could not hide the fact that he thought I was crazy to think about buying a fridge of all things before other far more important items. I had to agree with him; had I given the matter an ounce of consideration, I would surely have reached the conclusion that a bed ought to have been the first article to acquire for my new home.

'If this weather continues, a fridge is the last thing you will need,' he teased. 'These old stone cottages are freezing cold in summer, never mind in winter. You won't need to worry about the milk going sour, fridge or no fridge. Though come to think of it, during the winter a fridge will probably be useful for warming up the butter.'

'I don't suppose,' I began sheepishly, 'that you could help to transport this fridge from the shop to the cottage? Perhaps you know someone with a van who could do it for me?'

'No problem at all,' cried Spencer reassuringly. 'If it can wait until Thursday afternoon I can do it for you. I am free from two o'clock onwards.'

'Could you? That's great, thank you very much indeed.'

'Don't mention it, old chap . I'm happy to be able to help.'

CHAPTER SIX

By the time Thursday arrived, the weather had become atrocious. It was unbelievably cold and overnight there had been quite a heavy fall of snow. It was unusual to get snow in Luccombury at any time, and almost unheard of in November.

'This gets more and more ridiculous by the hour,' said Spencer good-humouredly. 'Ever since you ordered this blinking fridge, the weather has got colder and colder.'

'I'm not taking the blame for the weather but I have to say that I wasn't expecting it to be as cold as this. I was led to believe you didn't get much snow in the south.'

'We didn't before you came,' retorted Spencer. 'It's as if you brought it with you.'

I ignored the remark. 'Anyway, how are we going to carry the fridge? You know that it's packed in a large box which the shopkeeper said was too big to go into an ordinary car?'

I felt sure that Spencer would have an old van or a trailer that he used for transporting his cars; that was why I asked if he could help with the fridge.

'We'll tie it on the luggage rack on the back of the little Rolls.'

'On the luggage rack?'

'Sure. It's probably too big to go in the car, but it will be fine on the luggage rack. I've carried loads of things like that; it's a really useful way of transporting bulky items.'

The 'little Rolls', as he called it, was his beautiful green and black 1932 Rolls Royce saloon. It had no boot, but at the back was a steel-framed luggage rack.

'It should sit on there all right. You'd be amazed what I've managed to carry on that rack over the years. Jump in and we'll go round to the shop and collect it.'

I had never been in a Rolls Royce before and I felt extremely important. The seats were very comfortable but quite low down in the car; I could imagine that a short person would have difficulty seeing out through the windscreen. Like all old cars, it had that wonderful smell of leather. Spencer was wearing a cloth cap and scarf and looked very aristocratic as he lit his pipe before driving off. Progress was very slow. I'm not sure whether the car was incapable of going any faster, or whether this was the way Spencer usually drove. As the shop was not very far away it didn't take us long to get there, despite the snail's pace. There was no doubt that when we did arrive it was in style.

The box in which the fridge was packed was absolutely enormous; as the shopkeeper had warned. We tried to place it on the luggage rack but it was like trying to sit an elephant on a bar stool.

'We'll have to get rid of the box,' announced Spencer, ripping away at the cardboard. The amount of packaging seemed to be out of all proportion to the size of the fridge inside and it took quite a while to remove it. Eventually there was a huge pile of discarded wrapping, padding and packing, and beside it, looking quite tiny by comparison and standing naked on the snow-covered pavement, was my precious refrigerator.

'Why they had to put it in such a damn great box heaven only knows,' muttered Spencer throwing all the waste cardboard onto the back seat of the car. 'It should sit on the luggage rack now.'

It was certainly an improvement, but the fridge was still far too big to sit comfortably on the luggage rack. However, Spencer was determined not to be beaten.

'We'll pass ropes round it and tie it to the rear door handles,' he exclaimed suddenly, producing coils of rope from under the driving seat. 'That should stop it falling off.'

I was worried sick about damaging the Rolls. It seemed an utter desecration to treat a lovely vintage motorcar in this way, and I was beginning to feel guilty that I had asked for Spencer's help with the fridge. In fact, I was wishing I hadn't bought it. Spencer, on the other hand, was treating the whole thing as a challenge and did not seem the slightest bit concerned about the car.

'For goodness sake stop worrying. Cars like this are built like tanks. It's been used for worse things than this in its time, and no doubt will be again. There, the fridge looks pretty secure now. We'll have it round to the cottage in no time.'

He raised himself into the driving seat and relit his pipe before starting the engine. It seemed to turn over very slowly for several seconds before jumping into life. 'Right then, hold tight, Justin. Away we go. Keep an eye on the cargo to make sure we don't lose it on the way.'

In spite of the fact that Spencer referred to the car as his 'little Rolls', it was, in fact, quite a big and heavy vehicle. It glided away smoothly with nothing more than a whisper, producing great clouds of exhaust smoke, and negotiated the snow-covered road surface with no difficulty whatsoever.

We were making excellent progress and the fridge appeared to be held securely in place by the network of ropes tied round it. Suddenly, Spencer let out an excited cry and applied the powerful brakes in a manner which seemed to me to be far too fierce in view of the appalling weather conditions. Although we skidded for a full twenty yards on the icy surface, the car continued along a perfectly straight line, possibly because of its great weight. I was thrown violently forward and in most cars I would have hit my head on the windscreen but in this car the windscreen was so far away from the seat that I suffered no injury at all. Anxiously I looked behind and was relieved to see that my fridge was still in position on the luggage rack.

'Look over there' shouted Spencer with great excitement pointing furiously. 'Look, Justin, a badger.'

It was a wonderful sight. I had never seen a live badger before, and now there was one just a few yards away from us and he was apparently completely unperturbed by our presence. He was much bigger than I had imagined a badger to be from pictures I had seen, and he was scuttling along, nose to the ground, obviously with a mission in mind.

'I'll bet he's going to raid the dustbins in the yard behind those shops,' said Spencer. 'He's quite a large brock. Isn't he magnificent?'

'He's beautiful. I've never seen a live badger before. It's made my day.'

'There are lots of them around here. Foxes too. That's what living in the country is all about. There's so much wildlife to see and you'll be amazed at the enormous variety of birds that visit our gardens. It's one of the great perks of being in this part of the world. I absolutely love it, and I'm sure you will too.'

I was so thrilled to see the badger and Spencer's words made me think that moving to Luccombury had been a wise choice. I decided, however, that until I had sampled general practice dentistry, I ought not to jump to any conclusions.

We continued on our way and soon arrived at Ivy Cottage without further mishap, though quite a few people were attracted to the rather bizarre sight we presented. Many of the onlookers, it turned out, were patients of Spencer's, which was hardly surprising since his was the only dental practice in Luccombury. Many of them smiled and waved and, I suspect, were fairly used to Spencer's occasional display of mild eccentricity.

Very soon, the fridge was lifted from its perch on the back of the Rolls and, after much slipping and sliding on the icy path to the cottage, we safely installed it in the kitchen.

'Shouldn't cost much in electricity,' joked Spencer. ' There's absolutely no need to switch it on. Look, you can scrape ice off the inside of the windows. If I were you, I'd go and get some Arctic survival gear before you think of buying anything else.'

'You seem to forget,' I responded, 'that for the past six years I've lived in the north of England. This is nothing compared with what I am used to. You southerners don't know what real winter weather is like. I'd describe this as a bit on the cool side; nothing more than that.'

'Well I still reckon this place is an icebox. I wouldn't want to spend a winter in here myself. I think you'll find that southern winters can be surprisingly fierce. They're probably shorter than winters in the north, but we get our share of freeze-ups down here, make no mistake about it.'

As it happened, the next day was quite a bit milder and the snow quickly disappeared. Around midday the sky cleared and the sun shone throughout the afternoon with a surprising amount of warmth dispelling our fears that winter might be setting in early.

I decided to take a trip into Dorchester to have a look for furniture to fill my empty cottage. I discovered that buses from Luccombury to Dorchester and back were few and far between, and the journey took a very long time in proportion to the distance. In the end I decided to take the train. As I walked from the station into the centre of the town, I was again impressed by the general cleanliness of the streets and buildings and also by how much less traffic was on the road compared with a Friday in a northern city.

I wasn't really sure what particular items of furniture I was looking for. A bed was an obvious necessity, though I was finding it difficult to summon up much enthusiasm for wandering around furniture shops. Suddenly it crossed my mind that there were a number of second hand car dealers in the town, and the prospect of inspecting their forecourts to see what they had to offer made the outlook for the afternoon far more exciting. I had a strong feeling, however, that from a financial point of view it was probably not a very wise thing to do.

At the second garage I visited, I spotted something which made my stomach sink. I am not sure whether it was with excitement, or the fear that I was about to do something stupid. The object which caused the reaction was an Austin Healey Sprite in British Racing Green. It was in near perfect condition, or so it seemed to me at the time. The price? Well, let's just say that I would have to make another appointment with the bank manager to renegotiate my overdraft, but then he did say that he would be prepared to do so if necessary. I could only hope that he would look favourably on the purchase of a car. Anyway, the more I looked at the gleaming paintwork and the mirror-like chrome bumpers, the more certain I became that I had to own it.

Half an hour later, the deal was all sewn up. In a day or two I would be driving instead of walking. It had all happened so quickly but I felt sure that this was an opportunity not to be missed. I would have bought a car sooner or later, it was inevitable, but it just so happened that the right car had presented itself to me a little earlier than expected. I tried not to think about my overdraft and the fact that I would now be way over the limit. In fact, the cost of the car itself was enough to do that. But what did it matter? I now had a job and I would find a way of paying for everything; the road tax and insurance, and, of course, the furniture I needed for the cottage.

Surely my bank manager would realise that now I had stepped out into the big wide world, there would be certain items which were virtually essential.

CHAPTER SEVEN

Before I could take delivery of my new car, I had to think about arranging insurance. I had never owned a car before so I had never had a motor insurance policy and therefore had never built up a no claims discount. I had learnt to drive when I was eighteen and from time to time I borrowed my father's car, but I had never been in a position to afford a car of my own.

I had no idea how to go about getting the best deal so I looked in the Yellow Pages and phoned a few insurance companies. Two points quickly emerged. The first was that none of them was particularly excited about insuring someone in their mid-twenties with limited previous driving experience to drive a sports car, and the second point was that there were wide differences between the amounts I was being quoted by the different companies. I was hoping to get comprehensive insurance but I began to wonder if I would be able to afford it. The quotes I had been given were at least twice as much as I had hoped and expected to pay. Should I simply accept the cheapest and get it sorted out without further delay? At least then I would be able to go and pick up my car, or would it pay me to hold my horses and make a few more enquiries before diving in? It then occurred to me that Spencer must know something about motor insurance in view of the fact that he owned so many cars, and would undoubtedly be able to give me some advice.

'It isn't going to be cheap,' were his opening words. 'Insurance companies don't like young inexperienced drivers driving sports cars, and you don't have a no claims discount to help bring the cost down. My motor insurance is arranged through a patient of mine called Stanley Critchley. He runs some sort of insurance agency with his brother. I'm not sure if he is an actual broker, but he does the job of hunting around different companies to find the best price. I've been with him for many years now and he always seems to find me a competitive rate. I think he tends to specialise in finding cheap insurance for older drivers who are generally considered to be a better risk, but I'm not sure; he may be able to help you. I know he managed to sort out cover for the young chap who lives across the road. He's certainly under thirty but I would say he is more the type to spend his money on fast women and slow cars which, from a motor insurer's point of view, is a much more attractive proposition. Anyway, there's no harm in giving Stanley a ring to see what he has to say.'

It seemed a sensible idea, so I dialled his number.

'Hello.'

'Hello, I would like to speak to Stanley Critchley please.'

'He's not here. I'm his brother. What is it you want?'

'I wanted to speak to him about motor insurance.'

'Yes, that's his field of expertise. I deal with household and fire insurance, and he does the motor business.'

'When will he be there for me to speak to him?'

'Later.'

'How much later?'

'Can't say. I'm expecting him back sometime, but I don't know when.'

'Can you ask him to phone me when he gets in?'

'I could do but it's risky.'

'Risky? In what way?'

'There's a risk I'll forget to tell him.'

'Can't you write it down?'

'I could do but I might forget to give him the note. If I do remember to tell him, there's still a chance he'll get side tracked and forget to ring.'

'So you're saying that it's probably safer if I phone back later?'

'I reckon it is.'

'Okay. I'll ring again, but I would like to contact him as soon as possible because I'm desperately trying to arrange insurance on a new car I've just bought, and until I get it insured I can't pick it up from the garage.'

'Well, Stanley's your man if it's motor insurance you want to know about. What he doesn't know about it isn't worth knowing.'

'That sounds encouraging. I need to speak to an expert. I've phoned several insurance companies already and, to be honest, I am totally confused. I really don't know what to do for the best.'

'My advice to you is to do nothing until you have discussed it with Stanley. There are all sorts of traps you can fall into unless you know what you're doing. It is very important to get the right policy at the right price. That's our motto – "the right policy at the right price".'

'Sounds a good motto. As far as I am concerned I just want to get my car on the road with an insurance policy I can afford.'

'Price isn't everything in insurance – it's value for money. Lots of people make the mistake of choosing the cheapest policy. If they're unfortunate enough to have to make a claim, that's when they wish they'd looked a bit more carefully at the cover.'

'I'll remember what you said. Is Stanley likely to be in later this afternoon?'

'He could be, but you never really know with him. He's very much in demand and I know he had several people to see today. Best keep trying until you catch him.'

'All right, I'll phone back later. Thank you for your advice.'

I put the phone down with somewhat mixed feelings about Stanley Critchley's insurance agency. His brother had been pleasant enough but not particularly helpful, and there seemed a strong element of uncertainty about the whole thing which troubled me slightly. I was very anxious to sort out cover that day so that I could pick up my car without delay. I wasn't very happy about waiting around for Stanley to return to base so that I could contact him. Surely it wasn't asking too much for him to phone me when he got back. However, I obviously needed advice from an expert, and if it were true that 'what Stanley doesn't know about motor insurance isn't worth knowing', then I would be foolish to allow my impatience to prevent me from taking advantage of his knowledge.

I waited agitatedly until early afternoon. Maybe Stanley had gone back for lunch. I dialled the number just before two o'clock.

'He's not back yet. I haven't heard a word from him. He sometimes phones in, but he hasn't done so far today.'

'All right, I'm sorry to trouble you. I'll phone again later, if I may.'

I tried again at half past three without success and finally, at just after half past four, I managed to contact him.

'Stanley Critchley speaking,' came the welcome reply.

'Oh, Mr Critchley, I'm so glad I have finally managed to make contact with you. My name is Justin Derwent and I'm a dental surgeon. I've just come to Luccombury to work with Spencer Padginton. He suggested I phone you about arranging insurance for a car I've just bought.'

'Oh yes?'

'Yes. I understand that you're an expert in the field of motor insurance, and I would be very grateful for your advice.'

'I don't know about "an expert". I have been in the business for some time so I do know a thing or two about it. What are you looking for?'

'I'm looking for insurance cover, preferably comprehensive, on an Austin Healey Sprite I have just bought.'

'How old are you?'

' Twenty five.'

There was a sharp intake of breath at the other end of the phone, followed by a pause.

'How many claim free years of insurance do you have under your belt?'

'Well, I haven't had any accidents but I've never had an insurance policy before. This is my first car.'

There was another sharp intake of breath at the other end of the phone.

'Have you been convicted of a motoring offence?'

'No, never.'

'Well at least that's something. *I* wouldn't want to insure you in a car like that with your lack of experience, but then I'm not the insurance company I'm only the agent.'

There was another long pause. His next comment wasn't exactly inspirational.

'It might be possible to get cover at a price. I don't really know.'

'I thought you'd be able to give me some advice.'

'My advice is to buy a Ford Anglia.'

'But I've already bought the Sprite. Surely someone, somewhere will insure me?'

'They may do, I wouldn't really know.'

'So what do you suggest?'

'I suggest you get out the Yellow Pages and ring round some insurance companies to find the best quote.'

'Is that the best you can do for me, then? I was under the impression that it was your job to arrange insurance cover for people. Can't you at least suggest a company I could try?'

'I don't know of one that would be willing to give you cover – you're a high risk. But I can't know everything. Until you've phoned and asked, there's no way of knowing.'

I put the phone down in utter despair. So much for the notion that what he didn't know wasn't worth knowing. What was I to do now? I so badly wanted to get my car.

I went back to the notes I had scribbled earlier in the day when I had been trying to arrange insurance cover myself. When I spoke to the various companies on the phone, the situation hadn't sounded as hopeless then, as Stanley had made it appear to be. I had, in fact, found more than one company willing to take me on. Admittedly the premium was higher than I had hoped for, but right now the most important thing was to get a cover note so that I could pick up my car. I searched through my scribblings and found the name of the company that was offering the cheapest deal. Never mind what Stanley's brother had said as far as I was concerned, as long as it made it legal for me to drive the car I didn't care about anything else.

During the course of the year I could make some more enquiries and perhaps sort out a better deal when the time came to renew the policy. In the meantime, the premium would simply increase my overdraft a little bit more, that was all.

I cursed the fact that I had wasted so much time hanging on for Stanley's advice which turned out to be useless. I just hoped that the insurance company I decided to go with hadn't finished work for the day. I dialled the number and waited with bated breath to see if someone would answer. As it turned out, I was in luck and I gave them my details there and then. Quite by chance, they had a small branch office in Luccombury itself and it was arranged that I would call in the office first thing next morning to hand over my cheque for the premium and collect a cover note. I could then pick up my new car.

CHAPTER EIGHT

I was pleased that the snow had cleared away and not returned now that I was in possession of my new car. It was running beautifully and I was extremely proud to park it outside the practice when I arrived there on my first morning in the surgery.

I had moved into Ivy Cottage even though I still had not purchased any furniture. Ephraim had provided me with a table and three old chairs as promised, and Spencer had kindly given me an old camp bed. One of Ephraim's neighbours had donated an old wardrobe and a chest of drawers so at least I had somewhere to put my clothes. There was a built-in cupboard in the kitchen which I intended to use as a food store, but at present it was too dirty and needed cleaning out before it could be used for that purpose. I hadn't got around to it so far because I had been too preoccupied with my car. In the meantime, therefore, I used my new fridge as a storage cupboard. I hadn't switched it on because most of the food in there didn't need to be refrigerated, also, as the cottage was like an icebox anyway, anything that did need to be kept cold I simply placed on top of the refrigerator.

I decided that I would write to my bank manager to break the news to him about my car. I was not eager to meet him face to face and, as I was not going to be travelling back north at the present time, I thought that a letter was the best way to raise the subject with him. His reply came back with frightening speed and it was with considerable trepidation that I opened the envelope. Much to my relief, he did not seem at all concerned about my latest attack of extravagance. The gist of his letter was to state that whilst he was not prepared to extend my overdraft to cover the cost of the car, he was quite willing to offer me a loan so that I could make fixed monthly repayments over a period of three years. I was perfectly happy with the arrangement and immediately sent back the necessary forms duly completed.

I had to leave my pride and joy on the road outside the dental practice as there was nowhere else I could park it. This caused me some anxiety, though I tried to console myself with the fact that the road was reasonably wide at this point and approaching vehicles would have a clear view of the car. My concern for this helped to overshadow my understandable apprehension about meeting my first ever patients in general dental practice.

It was hopefully going to be a fairly easy morning. Spencer had been keen to book in patients to see me, but I had asked him to make sure that I would be given plenty of time with each patient until I found my feet. I was well aware that some dentists see a terrifying number of patients in a session, working at a phenomenal rate all the time, but I was not ready to do that just yet and I got the impression, though I had not yet seen it for myself, that Spencer didn't exactly overstretch himself.

I deliberately arrived early as there were lots of things still to be sorted out. During the previous week I had spent some time in the surgery trying to familiarise myself with the layout and finding out where everything was kept, but it would take some time before it all sank in.

Spencer greeted me and was obviously excited about something. 'Good morning, Justin. I'm glad you came early, as I've got something to show you. Come in here.'

I naturally thought it was some new piece of dental equipment he wanted to demonstrate to me and whilst I was interested, I was too preoccupied with the prospect of starting work to get too thrilled about anything new at that moment.

'What is it, Spencer?' I demanded somewhat grumpily. 'I need to get organised in my surgery before any patients arrive.'

'You've got plenty of time, there's no-one due just yet. You must come and see this first. What you are about to see has actually succeeded in getting Daphne out of bed before eight-thirty this morning. That is practically unheard of; she never gets up before eleven, and that's on a good day.'

There was a tinge of irritation in his voice as he spoke, but it was short-lived and his earlier excitement quickly returned. He led me through to the sitting-room where I found Daphne together with the most delightful little Dalmatian puppy.

'Come and meet Dotty,' Daphne called out. 'Spencer bought her for me yesterday. Isn't she absolutely beautiful?'

She certainly was beautiful. Highly playful with unlimited energy and needle-sharp little teeth. She was leaping in and out of the chairs, running back and forth from Daphne to Spencer so fast it made you dizzy.

'In a minute she'll flake out completely and sleep for a little while before the next burst of activity. Look out,' cried Spencer, 'she's going round in circles which means she's going to have a wee. Get her to the door, quick.'

The poor little soul was snatched up off the carpet and dumped unceremoniously on some sheets of newspaper by the door where she relieved herself as forecast.

'Just made it,' sighed Spencer smiling.

'She'll soon learn,' said Daphne, 'she's a bright little thing.'

'She's delightful,' I exclaimed as she rolled over in front of me so that I could tickle her tummy, 'but I really must go to my surgery and get ready for my patients.'

I was beginning to feel more nervous about my launch into general practice. I had wanted some time to unwind and quietly get myself prepared for the morning ahead. Dotty's frenzied activity had not had a relaxing effect upon me. Neither Daphne nor Spencer seemed to have any concern at all for my apprehension.

'Oh don't worry about it,' replied Spencer, 'you have loads of time before your first patient. There's no need to get yourself all worked up. It will soon be so routine you won't give it a second thought; general practice very soon becomes pretty boring.'

The Dean's words about general practice came flooding back to me, but at that moment I found it difficult to believe.

'Well, perhaps it does, but right now I cannot help feeling a bit nervous about it and I would like some time to get myself sorted.'

'Sure,' agreed Spencer, suddenly realising that he was being a bit thoughtless. 'You can come back and see Dotty later if you want to. Let's go up to the surgery now. I forgot to ask if you had any operating gowns. I thought I had better order some up just in case you didn't have any. I had no idea what type you prefer, so I ordered some like the ones I wear. You could have borrowed some of mine, but I don't think they would fit.'

I looked at his portly figure and was on the point of agreeing with him, then I thought better of it. I didn't want to be insulting, so I ignored the comment.

'No I don't have any gowns. I should have thought about it myself but thanks for ordering some for me.'

'Are these all right?' asked Spencer as he handed me a snow-white garment. 'Should fit, but try it on. I went for long sleeves rather than short. I hate short sleeves; you have to wash your arms. You haven't met Anna yet, have you? She only got back from holiday at the weekend. She's an excellent dental nurse; damned attractive too. Come to think of it, she should be working with me. I don't know why you should get the pretty one. Perhaps we'll swap and you can have Beryl.'

I had already met Beryl who I thought was a bit of an old dragon. She was in her mid-fifties and had worked at the Padginton Dental Practice for more years than anyone cared to remember. Spencer was, in fact, very fond of her. She was extremely loyal and, like all good receptionists, did an excellent job of protecting Spencer from the patients. She was kind but very firm and the long-standing patients of the practice knew from experience that they must not get the wrong side of her. Anna, on the other hand, had only worked there for about two years and was already working out her notice because she was leaving to take up 'proper nursing' as Spencer described it.

'It's a great shame she's leaving,' said Spencer. 'I've tried to talk her out of it but her mind is made up. I suppose you can't really blame her for wanting a more glamorous career than being a dental nurse all her life. I know Beryl has been, but there aren't many like her. I expect Anna will meet some bloke fairly soon and before you know it she'll be married with half a dozen kids. She's going to Chichester, of all places, to do her training. I ask you, Chichester; it's a Godforsaken place. Have you ever been?'

'No, I don't know it. When is she leaving?'

'In a month's time. You'll just about have got used to working with her. Never mind. I'll find you someone else when the time comes. Anna's glad you're starting work. She's found life a bit quiet since father retired; she got quite bored at times, I think. If you had started work here a few months ago she might not have thought about leaving. Still it's too late for that now. Oh, here she comes.'

Spencer introduced us and then went off to his own surgery.

'I'll leave you two youngsters alone together now, then. Anna will be able to show you everything you need to know. Try to keep your minds on the job.'

The glint in his eye told me exactly what he was thinking, and there was no doubt that Anna was very attractive. I was already sad that she would soon be leaving.

Thirty seconds later he poked his head round the door and said, 'If I were you I would sit Anna in the dental chair and have a practice run with that stool. You didn't do too well with it last time you tried.'

He disappeared again.

'Have you seen anyone use this stool?' I asked Anna.

'No, I haven't,' she replied. 'It looks extremely unsteady to me; I don't envy you perched up there all day.'

'It's not too bad once you're up there; it's getting on and off that's the risky bit. Shall we have a go before the first patient arrives?'

'You can,' she replied, 'I'm keeping well out of the way until you've gained some proficiency.'

I made a move towards the stool and was about to attempt to mount it when a sudden noise made me jump almost out of my skin. It was the front door bell, or to be more accurate, buzzer, which sounded like a chainsaw and was situated just outside my surgery door.

'Loud isn't it?' smiled Anna who was amused by my nervousness. 'Let's hope you get used to it before you stick the drill in someone's mouth. If you jump like that you'll slice their tongue in half.'

'Thanks for the encouragement. You don't fancy being my first patient then?'

'No I don't,' she retorted with a look of horror. 'You'll need about ten years' experience before I would let you treat me.'

She went to answer the doorbell, which she was able to do from just outside my surgery by means of an entry phone system.

She pressed a button, which allowed the patient to push open the front door.

'It's Mrs Godley, your first patient. Poor unsuspecting soul.'

'You're a great confidence booster, I don't think. I'm apprehensive enough without you making things worse.'

At that moment, Spencer appeared again.

'Your first patient is here. I thought it best if I were to introduce you to her. Would you go and fetch her, Anna?'

A few moments later Mrs Godley appeared. She was a formidable looking woman with a face like a tombstone.

'Ah, good morning, Mrs Godley,' Spencer began. 'I would like you to meet Mr Derwent. He is my new assistant and will be looking after you from now on.'

I held out my hand her but she ignored it.

'What do you mean, looking after *me?*' she boomed. 'I have been a patient of your father's for almost fifteen years. I assumed that when he retired I would become a patient of yours. I am certainly not prepared to put myself in the hands of some apprentice.'

'Mr Derwent is not an apprentice. He is very highly qualified. I am sure you will find him extremely competent.' Spencer assured her.

'I am not going to find out. I'm sorry Mr Padginton, but he looks like an apprentice to me. What experience has he had? Very little, I expect. I refuse to be told who is going to carry out my dental treatment. I will choose my own dentist, thank you very much. If you are not prepared to treat me yourself, then I shall go to another practice.'

Spencer refused to be intimidated by her.

'I am sorry,' he replied, 'but I have my own patients and I cannot take on any more. Mr Derwent is here to look after my father's patients. I have every confidence in his ability, and if you are not prepared to let him treat you, then you will have to go to another practice.'

'Very well,' growled Mrs Godley, 'but I think it is disgraceful. I have been loyal to this practice for fifteen years and this is how my loyalty is repaid. Mr Padginton Senior would never have behaved in this way; he was a gentleman. I shall find another dentist. Nobody is going to tell me what to do. I shall make my own choice.'

Anna showed her down the stairs and to the front door. Mrs Godley was still grumbling away to herself as she walked down the path.

Spencer turned to me. 'Silly old bat. Don't let it worry you, Justin. I expect that there will be other patients who feel like that; it's inevitable, I'm afraid. Father had some queer old sods on his books – he seemed to attract them – but hopefully not everyone will walk out on you. After a while they will accept you, but it is going to take time. Believe it or not, I had the same problem when I first started to work here. Nobody wanted me as their dentist, they all wanted to see my father.'

I thought it was very nice of Spencer to stand by me. It would surely have been easier for him to accept Mrs Godley as his own patient and I felt responsible for driving a patient away from the practice.

'She was a real old battle axe,' said Anna after Spencer had left us alone once more. She realised that the incident hadn't helped my confidence. 'Don't worry, they won't all be like her. I never liked her anyway. Old Mr Padginton was able to handle her, but she was always difficult to please.'

CHAPTER NINE

Because my appointment with Mrs Godley had been unexpectedly cut short, it meant that I had some twenty minutes to wait before my next patient was due. It would have been nice if my first encounter with a patient in general practice had not been quite so unsettling, and doubts as to whether or not I had made the right career choice came flooding over me. I realised, however, that there was no point in thinking too much about it. I had made my decision and it was a bit premature to be questioning whether or not it had been a wise one.

Anna was quick to spot that I had been upset by Mrs Godley, and she did her best to take my mind off it by asking me about my ways of working and what filling materials I preferred to use. There was a vast range available to dentists and they each had their own preferences. She asked me how I wanted them mixed and little things like whether I wanted her to stand close to the patient and hand the materials to me, or whether I preferred her to place them on the bracket table and leave me to get on with it, as Spencer did. It was a useful few minutes, and talking to Anna helped me feel a bit less demoralised by Mrs Godley.

'So who is my next patient?' I asked, trying to appear more cheerful.

'Mr Mauleverer,' Anna replied. 'He's not too bad; a bit inquisitive, but not malicious.'

'Let's hope I have more success with him than I did with Mrs Godley.'

'Don't worry about it,' said Anna comfortingly. 'It wasn't your fault.'

Spencer reappeared yet again, this time to introduce me to Mr Mauleverer who was a tall thin man in his seventies with snowy white hair and bushy eyebrows. He shook my hand warmly.

'Pleased to meet you, young fella. You've taken on a hard job following in old Mr Padginton's footsteps. He was a wonderful dentist, absolutely wonderful. There'll never be another one like him. Never mind, come on let's see what you can do; I believe I need a stopping.'

It sounded strange to me to hear a filling referred to as a stopping. It was not an expression that I had heard used in the north.

'Right, Mr Mauleverer,' I retorted, trying desperately to appear confident when in reality I was feeling anything but. 'Come and sit down and let me have a look.'

He sat in the dental chair and I slowly and carefully hoisted myself on to my revolving stool. I breathed a sigh of relief when I realised I was safely up there.

'I'll just lie you back now,' I said and pressed the appropriate button to recline the chair.

'Hey, hold on, young fella. You said sit, not lie down. Put me back up.'

'I'm lying you back because that is the way I was trained to work. Most dentists today operate with the patient fully reclined.' I explained.

'Mr Padginton didn't. I always sat upright for him.'

'But I work differently from Mr Padginton. In his day it was different, patients did sit upright then. Mine is the new system of working.'

'I'm sorry, but if it was right for Mr Padginton, then it's right for me too. I must insist on sitting upright whilst you treat me.'

'Very well, Mr Mauleverer, if you insist.'

I put the chair back into the upright position and looked into his mouth. His teeth were very worn down and some were broken. There was a great deal of heavy staining, which looked like tea stains. It wasn't immediately apparent to me which particular tooth he thought needed filling. I could have put forward a good argument for carrying out some restorative work on quite a few of them but obviously Mr Padginton had told him that one of them needed filling so I felt I had to go along with that. I decided that I had better check with the record card.

'Can't you find it?' demanded Mr Mauleverer, who must have detected my uncertainty.

'Just checking the charting, Mr Mauleverer.'

'It's this one up here.' He pointed to the upper left second premolar.

'Yes, I know that,' I lied, nevertheless grateful that he had saved me the embarrassment of having to admit I couldn't decide which tooth I should be treating. I examined it carefully and could see that it wasn't going to be an easy tooth to fill.

'It's quite a big hole, Mr Mauleverer. I think I shall probably have to put a couple of stainless steel pins in it to hold the filling in place.'

'Stainless steel pins,' he spluttered, 'whatever for? Mr Padginton's fillings always stayed in without the need for pins. No, if you put the filling in properly it will stay there without pins.'

'I'm sorry but the hole is so big. Without pins, the filling doesn't stand a chance. There isn't enough tooth left to hold it in place.'

'It seems to me that Mr Padginton just had the knack, which no doubt comes with experience. Probably when you have been in practice as long as he was, you won't need pins to hold your fillings in place. However, if you say it needs pins, then pins it must have, as long as it doesn't hurt.'

'You won't feel any pain,' I reassured him, 'because I'll give you an injection to deaden it.'

'An injection? Mr Padginton never gave me injections and he never hurt me once. I have always said the hallmark of a good dentist is one that can treat patients painlessly without injections.'

'That isn't always possible,' I protested. 'A pin has to be placed deep into the tooth and it can be sensitive. Even Mr Padginton would have found it difficult to do this painlessly without first giving an injection.'

'That's what you say, Mr Derwent, but I am sure that Mr Padginton could have done it. Comes with experience, I suppose. Anyway I don't want an injection. Just get on with it.'

'Very well,' I replied, rapidly becoming thoroughly sick of hearing how wonderful Mr Padginton was. I picked up the dental drill and began to move towards his mouth.

'Aren't you forgetting something , Mr Derwent?'

'Not that I can think of. What do you have in mind?'

'The er... what do you call it? Saliva rejector, I think Mr Padginton used to call it. He always used it. He used to clip it over my lip and under my tongue before he started drilling. To suck out the water, you see.'

'Yes I know what you mean. It's a saliva *ejector*. But didn't you find it uncomfortable?'

'Well, I suppose it was a bit, now that you come to mention it. Sometimes it would dig in quite painfully.'

'Precisely,' I said, feeling that this was the first point I had scored throughout the whole morning. 'I don't use that type of saliva ejector. Anna here will do the sucking out for you.'

'Well I don't know, Mr Derwent. I suppose I shall have to give it a try, but I can't help thinking that Mr Padginton's way was probably best. His experience over all those years would have shown him the most effective methods.'

I said nothing but started drilling. After about five seconds his hand shot up in the air like a schoolboy anxious to attract his teacher's attention. It narrowly missed my left temple. I stopped drilling immediately.

'What's wrong, Mr Mauleverer?'

'I just wanted to tell you that when Mr Padginton was drilling, he always said that if I wanted him to stop I must put up my hand. Will you stop if I raise my hand?'

'I just did, didn't I?'

'Yes, you did, but I just wanted to check. After all, your methods are completely different from Mr Padginton's – I am amazed just how different – so I couldn't be sure without checking. Carry on, young fella. You haven't hurt me yet, but I mustn't get complacent.'

I resumed the drilling. After another five seconds his hand shot up again. This time it was his right hand like a spring loaded lump of rock, and it landed with a sickening thud above my right eye. My head went back as if it had been struck by a thunderbolt. I saw stars and was very nearly knocked off my stool.

'I'm terribly sorry, Mr Derwent. I didn't mean to hit you,' came the abject apology.

'Don't worry about it,' I muttered, rubbing my head.

Anna found the whole thing highly amusing and was trying hard not to laugh out loud. I was beginning to feel slightly ruffled. He had already rubbed me up the wrong way by his constant comparisons with Mr Padginton, and I could see no reason at all why he had to wave his arms around in that ridiculous manner.

'I really am sorry, Mr Derwent, but Mr Padginton always used to stop drilling after five seconds to let me rinse my mouth. He used to count to five out loud so that I knew when he would be stopping. I was worried that you were going to drill on and on without a pause. I hate it when the water builds up in my mouth. Mr Padginton was most understanding about it.'

'Have a rinse now, then,' I replied sharply. 'I'll keep stopping for you, but can we get on?'

It seemed to take an interminable length of time to complete the drilling as his hand was continually signalling for me to stop. He wasn't content with just spitting out the accumulated water, but insisted on rinsing out several times at each break, head thrown back, shaking it from side to side. He used up at least five glasses of mouthwash.

Finally the drilling was finished and I even managed to drill the holes for the pins without hurting him. I was thankful for that and felt quite pleased with myself.

'That's all the drilling, Mr Mauleverer. We can fill up the hole now, I'll get Anna to mix up the amalgam.'

'You won't be stopping it today, though, Mr Derwent?' It came over more as a command than a question. 'Mr Padginton always put a dressing in first and left it in place for two to three weeks before he put in the final stopping. He was always most adamant that it was the right way to do it. I think it was to let the tooth settle down. Anyway I'm sure he knew what was best.'

'There's absolutely no need to put in a dressing,' I assured him. 'I can fill it up and finish the job right away. It will save you coming back.'

'I'm sorry, Mr Derwent, but I must insist that you do it Mr Padginton's way. After all, he had a great deal more experience than you.'

'Maybe he did, but I can assure you that there is absolutely no reason at all why I should not fill it here and now, and that is what I intend to do.'

'No, Mr Derwent, I won't allow you to do it,' he replied stubbornly. 'I don't mean to be difficult but I am sure that Mr Padginton knew best. Please pop a dressing in for me now and I'll make another appointment to see you in a couple of weeks.'

There was clearly no point in arguing with him any more. I wanted to stick to my guns and insist on doing things my way, but I decided that I would probably just make him annoyed. In any case, there didn't seem to be much chance of being able to bring him round to my way of thinking. In the end I meekly said, 'very well, Mr Mauleverer, we'll do it Mr Padginton's way if that is what you want.'

I dressed his tooth and Anna led him away to make another appointment. As soon as he had gone, Spencer appeared again.

'Did you have a hard time with him?'

'It wasn't all that easy. He wanted everything done exactly as your father would have done it. He also punched me in the face. He didn't mean to, but it was pretty painful, as well as humiliating.'

'I expect you will have put up with lots of patients comparing you to my father, but don't let it get you down. People will accept you in time. Now, on a far more important note, here is your daybook. I want you to list every patient you see and write down how much you earn on them at each visit. It is the only way to keep track of your earnings.'

'Well, there's not much point in writing Mrs Godley's name in there; I didn't even manage to sit her in the chair. How much did I earn on Mr Mauleverer?'

Spencer handed me a thick and very official-looking folder. 'Here is the list of National Health Service fees. Every item of treatment is listed. What did you do on him?'

'I drilled one tooth and placed two pins and a dressing in it.'

'Didn't you fill it?'

'He wouldn't let me. Said your father always dressed them first and insisted I did the same.'

'Then I'm afraid you don't get paid anything. The National Health Service only pays when you have actually filled the tooth. There's no fee for a dressing.'

I was completely incredulous.

'You mean that I went through all that, spent the best part of half an hour working on him, even got punched in the face and I don't earn any money for it?'

'Not a penny,' confirmed Spencer. 'That's the NHS for you. Believe me, it's by no means easy at times, and I dare say you will make a living once you get the hang of it, but you should have filled the tooth there and then.'

'I wanted to but, as I say, he just wouldn't let me. He claimed that your father always put dressings in first.'

'It's true that father did mess about a lot during his last few years, but then he wasn't so worried about earning money. He just liked chatting to people. The dentistry was of secondary importance. You must insist on doing things your way whether the patients like it or not, otherwise you will be working for nothing half the time.'

'I can see I have a lot to learn.'

'Yes you have, but you will learn quickly. Ah, I think Anna is coming with your next patient. I'm afraid this one isn't going to be easy either. She has been a patient of father's for about thirty years, so she isn't going to accept change easily. Still, you can only do your best.

'Good morning, Miss Morrison. This is Mr Derwent who will be looking after you from now on.'

I shook hands with her and she seemed quite amiable. I decided that it was probably best not to recline the dental chair too far. I gingerly lowered the backrest very slowly, waiting for her to object. Surprisingly she said nothing, though I did not risk taking her back more than a few degrees.

'You don't need any fillings,' I declared after a very slow and meticulous inspection of her teeth.

'That's good,' she replied looking quite pleased. 'You certainly gave them a very thorough examination.'

I began to feel pleased also, thinking that I was handling her well. I had the feeling that I was walking on broken glass and was desperate not upset anyone else that morning.

'I think perhaps I ought to give you a good scale and polish; you do have quite a lot of tartar, particularly behind your lower front teeth.'

'Yes, Mr Padginton always said I made a lot of tartar. He always cleaned them for me.'

I set about scaling her teeth, paying fastidious attention to removing every trace of tartar. I then polished them using lots of the polishing paste which most patients seemed to find particularly pleasant, probably because it had such a strong fresh taste. It took me far longer than I would have been able to spend if I had had a busy surgery, but at the end of it I was very happy to be able to send her away with teeth that were positively gleaming.

She thanked me and left the surgery with a smile on her face.

I was feeling very relieved and pleased that I had at last managed to treat one patient successfully, especially as Spencer had said that she might be difficult. Presumably I would actually have earned some money for the examination and scaling, though I wasn't sure exactly how much. I reached for the list of fees to find out.

Before I could open it, however, I heard her scream. She had walked only as far as the top of the stairs where there was a mirror. She had stopped to look at her teeth and wasn't at all happy with what she saw.

'Just look what a mess I am in,' she complained hysterically as she returned to my surgery. 'Look at my gums. They are bleeding, lacerated, torn to ribbons, ripped to pieces. Never in all the years that Mr Padginton treated me did he ever make my gums bleed. I have been butchered. I am losing so much blood I shall be anaemic! I thought I could taste it. I have never known anything like it before. What on earth were you thinking of to inflict so much damage on me? You aren't fit to practice dentistry, Mr Derwent. You are a butcher!'

She was working herself up into a frenzy. The colour had drained from her face and tears were streaming down her cheeks.

'Please calm down, Miss Morrison,' I pleaded. 'You won't become anaemic. I couldn't avoid making your gums bleed. The tartar on your teeth has irritated them and made them swollen and inflamed; they bleed at the slightest touch. It just wasn't possible to do a thorough job of cleaning your teeth without making your gums bleed a little. I haven't lacerated or torn them. You haven't been butchered. They will stop bleeding very quickly, and there is absolutely nothing to worry about.'

She was not convinced. 'You haven't heard the last of this, Mr Derwent. I am disgusted at the way I have been treated. You will be hearing from my solicitor. I shall certainly never allow you to treat me again. Mr Padginton was so gentle. Why did he have to retire? You haven't heard the last of this,' she repeated as she sobbed her way down the stairs.

'Not having a very good morning, are we?' chuckled Spencer who suddenly materialised on the scene. 'At least you can put something in the day book this time which, after all, is the main thing.' He said with a grin. 'You know this practice has quite a few patients I've been trying to get rid of for years without success. I am convinced now that you will have no difficulty at all in succeeding where I have failed. I must get them booked in with you.'

His eyes twinkled as he spoke and it was clear that he found the whole thing highly amusing. This eased my feelings quite considerably and I began to see the funny side of it.

'Your last patient this morning is new to the practice. I haven't seen him before. He phoned up first thing this morning because he has a problem, so Beryl put him in with you right away. You might have a bit more luck with him. There isn't much point in introducing him to you since I don't know him, so I'll leave you to it.'

'Hello, I'm Richard Darcy,' came a young man's voice, holding out his hand to me. 'It's awfully good of you to see me so quickly. I've broken a tooth and I'm worried sick it's going to start aching. I can't afford to have toothache in my job – I need to be on top form all the time.'

'I'm pleased to be able to help,' I replied, inviting him to sit in the dental chair. 'Your job sounds a bit like mine. I need to be in good shape. It's a difficult enough job when you are well, but when you aren't a hundred percent, it's murder. What do you do for a living?'

'I'm a solicitor here in Luccombury; in North Street. I've been here nearly three years now, ever since I left Oxford.'

'You used to work in Oxford, did you?'

'No, I mean Balliol College, Oxford where I took my Law degree.'

'Oh, I see. How do you like it here?'

'Very much indeed. Luccombury is a great place. The town itself is a bit quiet, but there's plenty of night life around without having to go too far. I have my own house and a new Opel Manta that goes like the wind. What more could you wish for?'

'Are you married?'

His face screwed up as if I had said something extremely unpleasant. 'Good God, no. Why buy a book when you can join the library? Are you married?'

'No I'm not,' I replied. His expression had shown such distaste that if I had been married, I would have felt almost embarrassed to admit it. 'I've only just come to Luccombury. I haven't been out of dental school very long. This is my first practice.'

'Do you know many people here?'

'I don't really know anyone yet,' I confessed.

'Well, perhaps you would care to join me for a drink one evening. I could show you some of the local night spots. You might like to see my new hi-fi equipment. I was lucky enough to pick up a pair of second hand Lowther loudspeakers. They take up a fair bit of room but the sound is incredible. You should hear the cannons in the 1812. My next door neighbour thought war had broken out! Mind you I was playing it at nearly full volume, and the amp delivers two hundred watts per channel.'

'Sounds fantastic, I'd love to hear it. Thanks for inviting me out for a drink – that would be great.'

'Okay, I'll ring you when I get back to my office and consult my diary. We'll fix up an evening.'

As a patient he was exceedingly apprehensive and very jumpy. I got the impression that he avoided dentists as much as possible and only really sought help when he had a problem. He did his best to cover up his anxiety by talking constantly. He obviously liked the look of Anna and openly flirted with her, trying to make her laugh, though this was probably borne out of nervousness as much as anything. When she picked up the aspirator tip and approached him with it, he said jokingly, 'what on earth do you intend to do with that? It looks like an instrument for procuring a miscarriage.'

I took the drill from its bracket and moved towards his mouth but he hadn't finished talking. He looked once again at Anna and the aspirator tip.

'In view of the possible alternative use for that instrument you are holding, I sincerely hope you have sterilised it well before using it on me. Are you sure you're qualified to use it?'

He laughed and Anna smiled back at him.

'I really think,' he continued addressing me this time, 'that you dentists have got it made. You are in the unique and most fortunate position of having the opportunity to get lovely female patients to lie out before you, and not only that, but somehow or other you seem to be able to recruit the most beautiful girls to nurse for you. I don't know how you manage it. Every dentist I have ever been to has had a really stunning nurse. Though I have to say that Anna here is probably the most gorgeous dental nurse I have ever seen.'

He turned towards her, looked her straight in the eye and said with a mischievous chuckle, 'I do really think you should show me your qualifications before we go any further.'

Anna remained impressively professional. She showed a restrained response to his comments, which helped to calm him down, but she refused to be drawn in too far. Eventually, in spite of his chatter and reluctance to be treated, I was able to repair his tooth.

When it was all over he looked extremely relieved.

'I can't begin to say how grateful I am to you, Justin, for seeing me at such short notice and for treating me so skilfully and painlessly; I am deeply indebted to you.'

He shook my hand and then turned to Anna.

'It has been a truly memorable experience to be comforted and so well looked after by such a delightful young lady. Your dental nursing skills are quite exceptional and it has been a real privilege to have received such wonderful attention. Thank you, my dear.'

He took her hand and kissed it and then edged his way backwards out of my surgery.

'I promise that I'll consult my diary as soon as I get back to the office and I'll phone you, Justin, to arrange an evening when we can go out together.'

CHAPTER TEN

'I really must do something about finding you a new nurse,' Spencer sighed with a note of urgency in his voice. 'Anna leaves in a week's time and I haven't even advertised for a replacement yet. I've been meaning to do it, but somehow I just haven't managed to get around to it. I've been so busy with the Sports Car Club business and the surgery has been quite busy too.'

'I hope you find someone with the right qualities for the job,' I replied.

'Oh, and exactly what qualities are they?' inquired Spencer suspiciously.

'How about blonde, about five feet seven tall, with...?'

'Never mind all that,' cut in Spencer. 'I'm looking for an old battle-axe who will keep you in check. And someone who will sort out the patients for you when they prove difficult.'

'Someone who will mother me, I suppose?'

'Exactly,' agreed Spencer. 'You leave it to me. I know what's best for you, and I reckon I am pretty good at weighing people up when they come for interview. My first impression is usually the right one. I'll find you a nurse. You don't want some dopey blonde who sits around all day painting her fingernails. I know just the type for you.'

'Anna isn't dopey. She is very efficient, in fact – a brilliant nurse – and they don't come much more attractive than her.'

'Well, she is very much an exception.'

Spencer had the tendency to be extremely pompous at times and I felt that this was one of those occasions.

'I'll phone the local newspaper office right away and see if I can get an advertisement in there in the next day or two.'

As it happened, Spencer was vaguely acquainted with the editor and managed to convince him of the urgency of the situation, with the result that the advertisement appeared the very next evening. He was surprised at the number of telephone calls he received in response and was quick to tell me that there had been an enormous amount of interest in the job and that finding me a suitable replacement would be no problem at all. However, he didn't continue to keep me informed of his progress with the matter, and when the day of Anna's departure arrived I still had no idea whether or not he had chosen someone.

I must admit that I felt I ought to have some say in choosing a nurse. After all, she would be working with me all the time and it was important that we got on well together. I thought Spencer was a bit mean when he didn't invite me to be present at the interviews. He made it quite clear that he would be the one making the choice and left me in no doubt that he thought that if it were left to me I would choose the wrong type of person for all the wrong reasons.

I was forced to accept the situation but I couldn't help showing a keen interest in how he was getting on. I decided to challenge him again on the subject.

'Have you had any luck in finding me a nurse yet, Spencer?'

'Don't worry, Justin. It's all in hand.'

'So you have found someone, then? I personally would have thought it would have been a good idea to get her to come in whilst Anna was still here to show her the ropes.'

'I was hoping to do that, but unfortunately it has not been possible,' said Spencer somewhat evasively.

'But you have found someone?' I persisted.

'Well I thought I had,' said Spencer even more evasively, 'but it didn't quite work out. Don't worry, you will have a nurse to help you on Monday. I'll guarantee it.'

He tried to keep all trace of uncertainty from his voice and if I hadn't been staring him straight in the face I might have been convinced. The way he turned his eyes away from me as he spoke, however, let me know that the situation was not as well under control as he was trying to make out. I would just have to wait until Monday morning to see what he had managed to sort out for me.

After work that afternoon, we all gathered together in Spencer's sitting room to say goodbye to Anna and to wish her well for the future. Daphne had baked some cakes and Spencer had brought in a vast quantity of his home-brewed beer. There was also sherry, port, gin, brandy, whisky, and about two dozen bottles of wine. In fact, there was enough drink for a party of fifty. Beryl was there and had managed to persuade her husband to join us. Even Mrs Duck, Spencer's cleaning lady, who normally only worked in the mornings had returned specially to see Anna and had brought her a huge box of chocolates.

Spencer's parents had been present for some time when Anna and I joined the party, and had already had a glass or two of wine. Anna had worked for Spencer's father prior to his retirement; he obviously thought a great deal of her and wanted to see her before she left.

'Anna, my dear,' he called out to her as we entered. 'You are looking very well.' He kissed her politely on the cheek and shook her hand. 'I hope you will be extremely happy nursing and I wish you all the very best for the future, but your leaving is a very serious loss to this practice and you certainly won't be easy to replace.'

'Thank you for your good wishes, Mr Padginton. I have been very happy here, but I do want to be a nurse.'

'I know you do and a jolly good nurse you will make too. I'm sure you are doing the right thing, but I do hope you will come back and see us occasionally to let us know how you are getting on.'

'Yes, I will. I promise.'

'And how are you settling in, Justin?'

'Oh, quite well thank you, Mr Padginton. Some of the patients are beginning to accept me now, but most of them think you were so wonderful they don't really want to be treated by anyone else.'

'When you have been practising as long as I was, you will have just as many patients who feel the same way about you. It takes time to build up relationships. Do you know, Justin, it doesn't matter how good or bad a dentist you are, there will be some people who think you are the best dentist in the world, and some who think you are the worst. The ones who like you tend to stick with you and over the years you collect quite a few of them.

It is inevitable, however, that you won't see eye to eye with everyone. Some people can be very awkward and however good you are, you are bound to upset someone once in a while. When you are dealing with the public, it's inevitable whatever job you are doing. It's not just dentistry. The fact that people are often nervous doesn't help, though. It can make some people act out of character so you must make allowances.'

Mr Padginton was a wise old bird and I felt somewhat comforted by his words.

'Anyway, changing the subject,' Mr Padginton went on, 'Spencer told me you are renting Ephraim Trivett's little cottage. How is it?'

'I love it. It isn't the warmest place on earth but it hadn't been lived in for some time. When I get the log fire stoked up it gets really cosy. I have only just about got the basic essentials to exist at present. It can't really be called civilised living, but I don't really mind.'

'They will all come in time.'

'Yes, I know. I'm in no great hurry, though. I'm having a telephone installed tomorrow morning at half past eight.'

'Very useful, especially for a single young man, though personally I can't wait to get away from the phone. The wife is rarely off it. Last year our private phone bill was twice as much as the practice phone bill. Can you believe it?'

'What's that, dear?' Spencer's mother, who was talking to Daphne, overheard the conversation and immediately came to join us. 'He does exaggerate so. I only use the phone when absolutely necessary. I can't help it if people phone me, can I?'

'But if others make the calls, dear, how is it they find their way on to my bill?'

'Well I don't know why our phone bill is so high. Perhaps there is a fault at the exchange. You ought to get them to check it out. I can honestly say I don't make many phone calls. In fact, I don't think I've made a single call for over a week.'

'You phoned your sister this morning.'

'Oh yes, I had forgotten about that one.'

'Last night you phoned Mrs Miller and Mrs Blackmore.'

'Well I had to phone them about the church flowers.'

'I don't doubt that you had good reason to call them, but they were still phone calls. You did actually also phone Mr Fraser, Mrs Campion, Mrs Stacey and, yes, Mrs Evans if I remember rightly. These are just a few of the calls that spring to mind which you have made in the past few days.'

'You must be checking up on me the whole time to remember all that,' snapped Mrs Padginton beginning to look really annoyed. 'I think it's a bit much I can't make a phone call or two without you making a note of it and throwing it back at me later.'

'I'm not throwing it back at you, dear, I am merely pointing out that you make more phone calls than you realise and that is why our phone bill is so high. I've known you spend two or three hours here chatting with Daphne and then as soon as you get home you are on the phone to her. It only takes two minutes to get home from here. Why can't you say what you have to say whilst you are with her?'

'It's because something else crosses my mind as soon as I leave. I can't help it. Women are like that.'

Spencer became aware of the increasing tension and quickly came over to ease the situation. 'We are here to drink Anna's health and wish her well for the future, not to start squabbling over domestic issues. Have some more wine mother and calm down.'

Spencer filled her glass and raised his eyebrows at me. He was very familiar with his mother's little peculiarities and knew exactly how to handle her.

Drink flowed fast and furiously for about two hours when Anna announced that regretfully she would have to leave because she was going to Chichester next day and had much to do in preparation. It was a nostalgic moment; everyone without exception was extremely sorry she was leaving. She had been an excellent dental nurse and a great asset to the practice, as well as a lovely person. At the same time no one wanted to stand in the way of her ambitions.

After we had seen her off I realised that I too ought to leave, as I had made arrangements for later that evening.

'You're not going are you, Justin?' said Spencer looking really disappointed. 'I was hoping we could make a night of it.'

'I'm sorry, Spencer, I have to go.'

'It's not a woman, is it?'

'No, it isn't a woman. It's Richard Darcy, a patient of mine.'

'You should never make friends of your patients or patients of your friends and if it isn't a woman then it isn't important,' said Spencer pompously.

'Oh shut up, Spencer,' Daphne cut in. 'If Justin has to go he has to go. Not everyone wants to drink themselves stupid like you do.'

'I'd love to stay, Spencer, but I have arranged to meet Richard. I can't just not turn up.'

'You could phone him up and tell him that something else has cropped up, or invite him here if you want to.'

Spencer looked so disappointed. I felt I would be letting him down if I left now. 'I'll phone Richard and make some excuse. I can always arrange to see him some other time.'

'Good show,' said Spencer brightening up. 'You know where the phone is.'

As it happened, Richard was quite relieved when I cancelled our arrangement because he said that he had had a particularly trying day and was suffering from a headache. By the time I had finished my phone call, Spencer had refilled my glass with more of his home brew. As I had already discovered, his brew was considerably stronger than pub beer and I could already feel the effects of it. The fact that I hadn't had anything to eat didn't help.

'Come on, Justin, drink up. The night is young. We shall be eating a little later. One of Daphne's friends and her boyfriend are coming. You will enjoy meeting them. She is a super girl; attractive too and her boyfriend is quite a character. He is a keen sailor. He has a thirty-foot sailing boat which he built himself, and the two of them have just sailed across the Atlantic in it.'

'Have they really? That's fantastic. I get seasick in a rowing boat on a lake in the park. There is no way I could do it even if I had the nerve.'

'I'd do it to be alone for a month with the lovely Carolyn,' said Spencer with a glint in his eye, then he checked himself because he thought that Daphne might be listening.

'Are you coming in to work tomorrow?' he asked loudly changing the subject.

'I haven't got any patients booked in, but I thought I might pop in to catch up with some paperwork. If I drink much more of this I doubt if I shall feel like it.'

'I should have arranged for Anna's leaving party to be before your Saturday on, not mine,' sighed Spencer suddenly realising that he had patients booked in. In fact it was going to be quite a busy morning.

'Bit of bad planning on my part,' he continued, 'though I must say this beer of mine doesn't seem to upset me as much as pub beer. The last time I had a really heavy session in a pub was the night before Christmas Eve two years ago. I went into the surgery on Christmas Eve morning feeling ghastly. The first patient was supposed to be having three fillings but I couldn't face that so I put in a dressing and sent him away, then I threw up in the surgery sink. I sat down for a while and tried to gather myself before seeing a second patient. I just about managed to put in another dressing, then I got Beryl to cancel the rest of the morning and I went to bed. I haven't drunk much pub beer since then. I think they must put some chemicals in it that disagree with me.'

At that moment the doorbell rang and Carolyn Stevens and Tom Cox arrived. Daphne went to let them in.

'Hello there,' Spencer called out. He immediately went over to Carolyn and kissed her. It wasn't just a brief peck on the cheek, he put his arms around her and held her tightly for as long as he dared bearing in mind that Daphne was close behind him. 'I'm so glad you could come.' He finally released her and shook hands with Tom. 'I want you to meet Justin, my new partner in crime.'

Tom was short and quite lightly built, but with a certain ruggedness which was enhanced by his deep suntan. He was very casually dressed in a clean but well-worn sweater and a pair of corduroy trousers. He smiled a lot and had a great aura of friendliness about him.

Carolyn also had a golden suntan, short dark hair and big soft brown eyes which twinkled as she spoke. She was wearing a very smart light grey trouser suit.

'So you're the one Spencer has hired to deal with all his geriatric patients while he looks after the dolly birds?' joked Tom offering his hand to me. 'Pleased to meet you.'

'Don't take any notice of him, Justin,' cut in Spencer, 'there's no truth in it. It's just that the old fogeys think I'm a bad-tempered, intolerant old misery, but they fall for Justin's youthful approach and fresh-faced appearance. I, on the other hand, seem to get on spectacularly well with the younger women. They probably go for my experience and maturity; look up to me like a father figure, I suppose.'

'Oh, just listen to him,' scoffed Daphne. 'Why don't you just admit you're becoming a dirty old man who likes having young attractive females stretched out in front of you, surrendering themselves to you?'

'Crikey, is that what it's like?' said Tom. 'I never realised that's what dentistry was all about. I reckon I should have been a dentist.

'Funnily enough, Richard Darcy – that's a new patient of mine – said that he thought dentists had it made because they have female patients lying out before them. He was quite envious about it.'

'What does he do for a living?' asked Tom.

'He's a solicitor,' I replied.

'They get enough perks of one sort or another; mostly financial I would say, judging by what I pay my solicitor,' said Spencer grumpily.

He fetched drinks for Carolyn and Tom and then filled my glass once more. By this time, I was beginning to feel distinctly unsteady on my feet and was sure my speech was beginning to slur. I decided to make a positive effort to slow down my rate of drinking.

'Where are you living?' asked Tom.

'In a little old cottage just on the outskirts of the village. It belongs to Ephraim Trivett. You leave Luccombury on the Dorchester Road and take the second turning on the left up a rough track. You go about a hundred yards and there is a little group of cottages.'

'Is it the one covered with ivy?'

'Yes, that's the one.'

'Oh yes, I know the cottage. Lovely old place. It hasn't been lived in for some time, has it?'

'No, that's right. It was a bit damp at first but it's slowly drying out now. Where do you live, Tom?'

'I live out in the sticks,' he replied. 'I have a bungalow about a mile and a half south of Luccombury. It's up a winding track tucked away in the trees. If ever you come to find me, bring a flask and sandwiches with you because you can quite easily get lost and be missing for days.'

'Sounds lovely.'

'It suits me,' Tom replied, 'though I haven't been there much recently. I've just come back from America.'

'Yes, Spencer told me. You sailed there and back on a small boat, didn't you?'

'It wasn't that small. Thirty-six feet to be exact.'

'Sounds small to me but then anything smaller than the Queen Elizabeth is small as far as I am concerned.'

'You're not a sailor then?' said Tom.

'No, definitely not. I like to keep my feet firmly on dry land.'

'What do you do when you aren't gazing into people's mouths? Do you have any hobbies?'

'Yes, drinking,' Spencer chimed in smiling.

I ignored the remark and carried on talking to Tom. 'To be honest I haven't really settled into normal life yet. I only left university two months ago, and as I've been living on a grant for the last six years, I didn't have any money to spend on anything other than books and food. Now that I'm working, I intend to buy myself a decent camera. It's something I've always wanted.'

'Funny you should say that,' Tom replied. 'I always promised myself a good camera and I finally bought one just before I left for America. I have started developing and printing my own films. It's really interesting.'

'I'd like to do that.'

'You must come and see my darkroom and you might like to come to the Luccombury Camera Club. I joined as soon as I came back to England. It's a great way to learn about photography.'

'Yes, I'd like that. I don't really know at the moment what sort of camera would be best for me.'

'There are plenty of people at the club to give you advice. They meet on Monday evenings. If you want to come, give me a ring on the Sunday evening before and I can arrange to pick you up.'

At that moment, Daphne announced that food was ready for us in the dining room, which was in fact also the patients' waiting room. It looked quite different now that the furniture had been rearranged and the magazines removed. The table had been extended to seat all of us and Daphne had certainly been busy in the kitchen preparing what turned out to be a marvellous meal. Spencer was wine waiter and kept a constant watch on our glasses to make sure they were kept filled at all times. I was almost frightened to take a sip because as soon as the level of wine in my glass dropped, Spencer immediately topped it up again. It made it very difficult to know exactly how much one was drinking, and I felt a great need to slow it down.

He was in fact quite a wine connoisseur and had matched the wines to the various dishes quite admirably, though I was beginning to reach the stage where the taste didn't seem to matter anymore. I tried to tell him that I had just about drunk enough but he refused to accept that this was so and assured me that a little more wine would not do me any harm at all. By the time we got to the cheese and biscuits I had reached that most dangerous state when common sense with regard to alcohol had more or less deserted me.

Spencer went to each of us in turn, offering port or brandy. He was distinctly glassy eyed himself now and when I asked for brandy and held out a wine goblet instead of a brandy glass, he filled it to the brim with his finest five star cognac.

I can remember drinking it down as if it were fruit juice, but quite honestly I can remember very little else after that. I don't know how long the party went on for. I can't remember saying good night and leaving Spencer's house. What is more frightening is that I cannot remember anything at all about my journey home.

CHAPTER ELEVEN

The sudden, ear-splitting, piercing shrillness of a metallic bell jerked me back to a state of semi-consciousness. I was lying on the sofa in the sitting room, which one of the neighbours had given to me only a day or two ago. I was still dressed. It was already daylight and a pure reflex action caused me sit bolt upright. I couldn't believe how bad I felt.

Where the hell am I and what on earth was that bell? Christ, there it is again. I winced, holding my hands up to my ears to try to exclude the penetrating noise which felt for all the world as if it were causing my brain to rattle against the inside of my skull.

Doorbell, came the gradual realisation. Who on earth could it be and what was the time? What day was it? What was I supposed to be doing today? Am I working? Why am I not in bed? Of course, I remember now; they've come to install the telephone.

I leapt to my feet. Unfortunately the abrupt change of position was too much for my delicate condition and I promptly passed out. As I went down I cracked my head on a chair just to add to my problems. When I came to, my head was pounding like a steam hammer. My ears were ringing, my tongue felt like a piece of leather, and my stomach felt as if it were inside out. I don't know how long I was unconscious. It was probably only for a few moments and the persistent ringing of the doorbell let me know that whoever it was outside was still there. I dared not risk trying to stand up again, so I crawled on all fours to the door. Heaven knows what the telephone engineer thought when I finally managed to open it. Frankly I felt too bad to care.

'Are you all right?' he began.

I can remember thinking, 'what a stupid question. Do I look all right?' However, I am pleased to say that I remained polite.

'Yes, I'm okay. Don't take any notice of me. I'll be fine in a minute.' I groaned, hoping that death would come before long and put an end to my misery.

'Where do you want me to put the phone?' he asked dropping his bag of tools with a resounding thud, which hurt just as much as if he had dropped it on my head.

'Anywhere will do; wherever is easiest,' I replied, unable to gather up enough brainpower to think about it.

'I'll put it here then, if that's all right with you.'

'Fine,' I muttered, 'fine.' Then I crawled back to the sofa and slumped back into a semi-comatose state. I have no idea how long the engineer was there. My next recollection was of him standing over me trying to wake me up to let me know that the job was finished.

'Thank you,' I managed to utter feebly. 'Thanks very much.'

'Are you sure you're all right? Can I get you a doctor?'

'No, I don't need a doctor. I just had a very heavy night last night. I'll be better soon. Can you see yourself out?'

'Yes, don't worry about me. You take it easy. Hope you feel better soon. Goodbye.'

I dozed for about another half an hour after he left, then I managed to rouse myself sufficiently to drag myself to the newly installed phone. I wondered if it would be working yet. I picked up the hand piece and, to my great relief, I heard a dialling tone.

'Hello Spencer, is that you? It's Justin here. I feel absolutely awful. I won't be able to come in this morning. I'm sorry.'

'I can't say I'm surprised. I feel a bit under the weather myself, but it was a good evening, wasn't it?' said Spencer.

'Yes, it was,' I replied meekly, thinking that I was certainly paying a heavy price this morning for last night's enjoyment.

'I'm relieved to know that at least you are still alive, though I must say that I think you were a bit reckless with the brandy. You really ought to drink a little more responsibly you know, Justin.'

'Come on, Spencer, you were the one who filled up my glass.'

'I don't remember that. I think you are mistaken. I certainly wouldn't dream of forcing drink on to someone who didn't want it.'

I wanted to point out that it was he who persuaded me to cancel my evening out with Richard Darcy so that I could stay and drink with him and that he kept on filling my glass with wine all through the meal before giving me that huge glass of brandy. However, I felt too ill to argue with him.

'Don't worry – you stay at home and look after yourself. Some of us have to carry on, but that's fine, I can cope. Give me a ring if there is anything you need. I'll see you on Monday then, Hope you soon feel better.'

CHAPTER TWELVE

'Feeling any better?' Spencer called out as he heard the front door close behind me.

'I'm all right now, thanks but I can't ever recall feeling quite so bad. I never want to see, smell or taste alcohol again. I've learnt my lesson once and for all.'

'That's what we all say until the next time. You'll no doubt do it all over again some day soon.'

'Not for a very long time.'

'Did you have a good weekend?'

'No, not really. It took until about four o'clock on Sunday afternoon before I began to feel half normal. How was your weekend?'

'It was quite good. I managed to do a lot of work on my car and I am pleased to be able to tell you that I've found you a new nurse. I said I would, didn't I? Though I don't think you believed I would manage it.' He sounded extremely smug as if it had been a major achievement.

'Really? What's she like?'

'You'll have to wait and see. She should be here very shortly, I told her to come early.'

'Has she any previous dental nursing experience?'

'Well, no, but I am sure she will soon pick it up. In any case, that could be an advantage. You will be able to mould her to your way of working. You will start with a completely clean slate; she won't have picked up any bad habits, so to speak.'

'How old is she?'

'Not quite as old as I would have liked'

'Well, how old?'

'About twenty,' replied Spencer quietly.

'Twenty!' I spluttered in amazement, thinking that things were sounding a bit more promising. 'I thought you wanted a mature woman. You always said you didn't like young nurses. You wanted someone old enough to be able to keep me in check.'

'I know, but unfortunately we didn't have any mature applicants. I am sure the one I have chosen will be perfectly suitable. She seems a very nice girl, very quiet and respectable, and not too ...' He paused as if searching for the right word. 'Well, not too ostentatious.'

'What exactly do you mean by that?' I demanded, suddenly thinking that my earlier burst of excitement had probably been a bit premature.

'I'm not saying any more about her. You will have to find out for yourself.'

'I can't wait,' I replied somewhat sarcastically, though I did think to myself that a twenty-year-old did sound infinitely preferable to the old battle-axe I had been expecting. 'By the way, do you know Dr MacKean?'

'Balfour? Oh yes everybody knows Balfour MacKean; he's been practising medicine around here for about a hundred years. Why do you ask?'

'I have an appointment to go and see him for an insurance medical. You remember the insurance rep came to see me last week? He suggested that I should increase the cover on my sickness insurance policy. He gave me the impression it would be perfectly straightforward and that it would all be arranged without any problem at all. It now appears that they won't do it without a medical examination. I hate medicals. In fact, I wouldn't have bothered to increase the cover if I had known.'

'MacKean is all right. He is a Scotsman, and like all Scots is a bit on the mean side. He doesn't believe in spending money. His surgery is apparently a bit antiquated, or so I've heard,' said Spencer with a grin.

I thought to myself that Spencer was a good one to talk about antiquated surgeries when you considered what his was like.

'I've heard that some of his methods might be a bit out-dated,' Spencer continued. 'He still believes in leeches and thinks that amoxicillin is some kind of rocket fuel. But he is a very likeable old chap. I would rather go to him for an insurance medical than to some young whippersnapper. I shouldn't think his examination will be too searching. As long as you don't have to be carried into the surgery and you've got a pulse, you'll be passed as fit.'

Just as Spencer finished speaking the front door bell rang. 'That could be Sandra,' announced Spencer sounding excited, or was it apprehensive? He ran to the door.

'Hello there, my dear, do come in.' I heard him say. There was no doubt in my mind now that there was a distinct note of apprehension in his voice. 'Justin's in here.'

I don't quite know what I had been expecting from what little Spencer had told me about Sandra, but when I saw her I was surprised. She was a frail little mouse-like creature with vivid ginger hair and freckles.

'Hello, Mr Derwent,' she began, holding out her hand and trying to force a nervous smile.

'Hello, Sandra, nice to meet you,' I returned, somewhat taken aback by the formality. I almost told her that it was in order for her to use my Christian name, but then decided that perhaps it wouldn't be a bad thing to limit familiarity at this stage.

'I must try and find you an overall to wear,' said Spencer, 'I imagine that Anna's would be too big for you. Daphne was supposed to be looking some out for you. I don't know whether she did or not. She's still in bed at the moment and not likely to be up before twelve.' He looked at me as he spoke and I knew what he was thinking.

'I'll go and see if I can find something for you.' He departed, leaving us alone together.

'What was your last job, Sandra?' I asked in an attempt to break the ice as well as out of interest.

'I haven't done very much, really. I worked on the check-out in a supermarket for a while, then I helped my father who's an insurance broker.'

'Why didn't you stay on with him? Didn't you like the work?'

'No, not very much. I wanted to be a nurse, really. You know, a proper nurse in a hospital but I don't think I'm clever enough. I thought dental nursing might be the next best thing.'

'It's hard work, you know. People can be quite difficult to deal with which can be very trying, and the job is also physically demanding. You'll find you walk miles in a day going to answer the door and the telephone.'

'Answer the telephone? I didn't know I'd have to do that. I hate the telephone. Mr Padginton never told me I'd have to answer the telephone. That's the main reason I hated working in my father's office because he wanted me to deal with clients on the phone.'

'Don't worry, you'll get used to it.' I reassured her. 'I don't expect you'll be doing it for a while anyway, until you're more sure of yourself.'

'I hope not. I do hope not. The idea of answering the phone terrifies me.'

'This is the smallest overall I can find,' said Spencer, suddenly appearing. 'Try it on.'

Small though it was, it looked like a bell tent on Sandra's tiny frame. It came down almost to her ankles and would easily have gone right round her twice.

'It'll do,' announced Spencer.

I think Sandra felt a bit ridiculous in it, so I tried to boost her confidence.

'It's fine. You need something to protect your clothes; it can be very messy.'

'Why don't you take Sandra to your surgery, Justin and show her round before the patients start arriving?' Spencer suggested.

'Sure, come on Sandra.' I responded, leading the way.

'Mr, er, Derwent...' Sandra stammered as if she had something pressing to say to me but felt afraid to come out with it.

'What is it, Sandra?'

'Will there be a lot of, er… a lot of ... er ...well, blood?' Her nose turned up and there was a look of horror on her face as she said it.

'Why do you ask? Does it worry you?'

'I can't stand it. I shall pass out, I know I shall. I do hope there won't be any this morning.'

'Well things can get a bit bloody sometimes,' I replied somewhat harshly, thinking that there was no point in lying to her. 'You'll get used to it. A lot of people feel a bit squeamish at first. Even one or two of my friends at university, who went on to become dentists, passed out in the early days.'

'I couldn't stand it,' she exclaimed, working herself up into a state of panic. 'I really couldn't stand it. There's no way that I could ever get used to it.'

'Don't worry,' I returned hastily, trying to prevent her from getting too upset. 'We'll break you in gently. You'll be amazed how quickly you will become accustomed to it. Try not to think about it now; let's just take one step at a time. Most of the time we'll just be doing fillings and making dentures. There are a lot of people around here who haven't got any of their own teeth left.'

'Dentures! You mean false teeth? Ooh, I won't have to touch anybody's false teeth, will I? Ugh, I couldn't bear to do that, I'd be sick on the spot, I know I would. I think I'm going to be sick now just thinking about it.'

'Calm down,' I exclaimed, wondering how Spencer could possibly have thought she would be any good as a dental nurse. 'You won't actually have to touch any false teeth. All you will have to do is to hold out a bowl so that they can drop their dentures into it. That's all.'

'I don't know if I can even stand the sight of them without being sick. I hate false teeth.'

'Just forget it at the moment. It'll be all right as long as you don't work yourself up into a state. Let's concentrate on some of the materials we'll be using. It will be your job to mix them for me.'

'I think I might be able to manage that,' said Sandra brightening up a little.

'Good. I'm sure you won't find it too difficult.' I was somewhat relieved to think that we had at last found a glimmer of hope.

I demonstrated to her how to mix amalgam filling material which she seemed to grasp without any problem. She was noticeably encouraged by her achievement and started to look a lot happier. I was about to show her how to fill the carrier so that we could place it into a tooth and what her role in the operation would be, when the buzzer outside my surgery door sounded indicating that a patient had arrived. It startled Sandra so much that she jumped about a foot in the air and let out an ear-piercing screech. As she did so, she threw the pot of amalgam we had just mixed up into the air.

'It's only someone at the door,' I explained. 'It takes you by surprise until you get used to it. If it were any quieter you wouldn't be able to hear it over the noise of the drill. Go to the entry phone and see who's at the door.'

Sandra hesitantly shuffled over and picked up the handset.

'Who is it?' She whispered so quietly that the patient at the other end could not possibly have heard her. She waited anxiously for a reply which didn't come. After a few moments the patient obviously concluded that his first press of the bell was not producing any response so he pressed it again, this time more persistently.

Unfortunately for Sandra, the sound of the buzzer emanated from the earpiece of the handset, which was tightly pressed against her ear. She let out a second shriek considerably louder than the first, dropped the handset and clasped her hands to her head. Beryl heard the commotion and promptly came to the rescue.

When Sandra had regained her composure, I thought I ought to give her a brief lesson on answering the doorbell.

'You must speak loudly and clearly, or the patient won't be able to hear you, and I don't think it sounds very welcoming to say "Who is it?" What you should say is "Good morning, can I help you?", preferably in a cheerful voice. Anyway, it is Mr Hitchcock who has just arrived; he is our first patient. Go and fetch him from the waiting room.'

Sandra disappeared and a few moments later returned followed closely by a somewhat bombastic looking, round, little woman. Some considerable distance behind her trudged her rather disgruntled and henpecked looking husband.

'Good morning,' blasted the woman.

'Good morning,' I retorted, becoming immediately aware that Mrs Hitchcock intended to take command of the situation.

'Come on, Harold' she snapped. 'The dentist hasn't got all day. Get in there and sit down.'

Harold's face lacked any sort of emotion and he said nothing as he made his way very slowly and deliberately to my dental chair.

'Good morning, Mr Hitchcock and what can I do for you?'

'It's his teeth,' barked Mrs Hitchcock.

'Well yes, I thought it might be,' I replied sarcastically, beginning to feel great sympathy for the poor little man who appeared to be totally overwhelmed by his domineering wife. 'Can you be a bit more specific?'

'It's his teeth,' repeated Mrs Hitchcock. 'His false teeth; they're no good. They won't stay in his head. Every night he falls asleep in front of the television, his mouth drops open and down comes his upper set. It looks horrible. And when he yawns and his bottom set lift up and his top set drop it nearly makes me sick.' She screwed up her face, groaning and shaking her head, then she put her hands to her face closing her eyes in utter abhorrence. It was an Oscar-winning performance and left me in no doubt that, at least as far as she was concerned, the situation was desperate.

'I can't stand it any longer. It's driving me up the wall. You've got to do something to keep them in.'

'How long has he had them?' I began, then suddenly thought that I ought to be addressing my question to Mr Hitchcock who so far hadn't said a word. 'How long have you had them, Mr Hitchcock?'

Mrs Hitchcock immediately jumped in. 'Must be ten years. It was soon after our Elsie's wedding, that's my sister, and that will be eleven years ago next month. You should know anyway,' she said with some venom. 'You should have the records. Old Mr Padginton made the teeth. Don't you keep the records?'

'Oh yes, we do have the records,' I declared picking them up and scanning through them. 'You are almost right. Mr Padginton made the dentures twelve years ago.'

'No, that can't be,' insisted Mrs Hitchcock, 'I'm sure it was after Elsie's wedding. Don't you remember, Harold? I said to you at the reception that your teeth were clicking whilst you were eating the wedding cake. It was so loud everybody was looking at you. I said then, that as soon as the Whitsuntide holiday was out of the way you would have to go and get your teeth seen to. I told you. You must remember?'

Harold looked completely blank for a few seconds then broke his silence with a definite 'No'.

'What do you mean, no? Don't be ridiculous – of course you remember. There's no way I could possibly forget. I have never been so embarrassed in my life. It sounded absolutely awful, you clicking away like that.'

'You are always saying my teeth click. You said it about my last set and the ones before that, and now you say it about the ones I've got now. I can't hear it.'

'Well you wouldn't, would you?' boomed Mrs Hitchcock. She turned towards Sandra who was quivering in the corner of the surgery looking terrified. 'I'm sure he does it deliberately to get me worked up,' she ranted on. 'He takes great delight in getting me annoyed. He knows I've got high blood pressure and I'll swear he's trying to kill me off with worry.'

She looked back at Harold with venom in her eyes. 'Come to think of it, you never did like our Elsie. Oh, you never actually said so, but I could tell. You never wanted to go to the wedding, you were really put out because it was the day of the Grand National.'

Turning to me this time, she said, 'horse racing and his allotment – that's all he can think of. I wouldn't mind, but every horse he backs always loses and he never grows anything worth eating. If you ask me, he was deliberately clicking his teeth to annoy me and everyone else at the reception as a sign of protest. Well, I can't put up with it any longer and now that they're dropping down as well, you've got to do something about it.'

'Let's have a look at them, Mr Hitchcock,' I said, trying to put a note of optimism in my voice in order to create the impression, with Mrs Hitchcock at least, that I might be able to help. In truth, I had a gut feeling that I too was backing a loser. I adjusted the operating light and slowly carried out a long and extremely thorough examination of his mouth and dentures. Mrs Hitchcock sighed impatiently, but I was not going to be hurried. At least they wouldn't be able to say that I had rushed through the examination.

'They are a bit loose aren't they?' I declared finally. As soon as I said it I thought it might have been wise to think of something a little more erudite to say. 'The back teeth are very worn down and they don't meet very well now. It must be difficult to chew with them. How long did you say you have had them?'

'I just told you,' blurted out Mrs Hitchcock, 'ten years.'

'Oh, yes, you said. It's just that they look a lot older than that.'

'Well, they're not.'

'Actually,' said Harold sheepishly, 'I could never wear the last set Mr Padginton made for me, so I went back to wearing the previous set.'

I thought Mrs Hitchcock was going to explode. 'So you're saying that the teeth you're wearing aren't the last set you had made? No wonder the damn things won't stay in your head – they must be twenty five years old! You never said you couldn't wear the new ones. After all the money we paid for them! If you couldn't wear them, why didn't you go back with them and get them sorted or get your money back?'

'I didn't want to make a fuss. Mr Padginton had done his best. It's just that the old ones were so comfortable. I don't really know why I went for new ones.'

'That's Harold for you; too pathetic to go back and complain,' said Mrs Hitchcock, addressing her moans in Sandra's direction once more.

I decided to try to continue with the examination. 'Can we take them out so that I can have a look at your gums? Sandra, bring that small stainless steel bowl over here, please.' Sandra's face drained of all colour as she picked up the bowl and held it out to Mr Hitchcock at the fullest extent of her outstretched arm. She had her eyes tightly shut and the expression on her face was as if she were being presented with a dead rat. She winced as Mr Hitchcock's dentures clattered into the bowl. Immediately she banged the bowl down on to the worktop so hard that the dentures nearly jumped out. She then went to the sink and furiously started to wash her hands.

'Your gums look quite healthy,' I announced after a thorough inspection, 'though they have shrunk somewhat since those dentures were made, but that's to be expected in view of the length of time you have had them.'

'My gums feel fine,' confirmed Mr Hitchcock and his wife grunted. 'I can eat perfectly well with them; they don't hurt or anything. I can't see what the fuss is about. I wouldn't be here at all, but the wife insisted.'

'Well,' I said, 'it is true that your gums have shrunk and the dentures don't fit as well as they used to, but the changes will have occurred very gradually over a period of time and you have adapted so you aren't aware of the changes.'

'As I said, they feel fine to me.'

'Shut up, Harold,' called out Mrs Hitchcock, 'you're talking rubbish. You have come here to get something done to make sure your teeth stay fixed in your mouth. If you don't have something done with them, you needn't bother to come home, because I can't stand to watch you asleep in front of the television with your teeth hanging out any longer.'

Reluctant as Harold was to have any treatment, Mrs Hitchcock was definitely the boss and it seemed that I was going to have to try to satisfy her demands.

'I think the time has probably come for you to have a new set of dentures,' I declared finally, thinking that this would probably be what Mrs Hitchcock would be wanting. Unfortunately I was wrong.

'New dentures? I'm certainly not paying out for any more. He says he can wear these and they are comfortable, so all he needs is for you to tighten them so they don't drop down, and then we shall all be happy. You need to put in a lining to take up the slack so that they grip his gums. That's all that's needed.'

'I don't think that relining them would be the complete answer, Mrs Hitchcock. You see, the back teeth are almost worn completely away and the bite isn't very even any more. I do think it will be necessary to make completely new dentures.'

'I'm sorry, but he's not having new ones. He must put up with the worn back teeth. He doesn't have any trouble eating. If you saw what I pack him up for his lunch every day! I don't know where he puts it. I'm forever cooking and baking. He gets queer if I don't bake a fruitcake every week. He gets real nasty with me. Don't you worry, he can eat all right. I wouldn't mind, but look at him – thin as a rake. Anybody would think I starve him.'

Looking at the formidable Mrs Hitchcock and her meek little husband, I found it difficult to visualise him 'getting nasty with her', as she put it.

All this time, Sandra was standing motionless, as white as a ghost and without any sign of emotion. She was as far away from Mr Hitchcock's dentures as she could get without actually leaving the room.

'Well, Mrs Hitchcock, my professional opinion is that new dentures are needed. The ones he is wearing are worn out and beyond the point when relining would be beneficial. My advice is that it would be a waste of time and money to try to do anything to improve them.'

'I don't see why we need to do anything,' chimed in Harold. 'They are my teeth, after all, and I am perfectly happy with them. As far as I am concerned, there is nothing wrong with them.'

'I think we must accept what your husband says.' I responded. 'You say he needs his dentures relined, I say he needs new ones, and he says he is happy with them as they are. The final decision must be his. As one of my tutors at university, a Yorkshire man, used to say, "when in doubt, do nowt". I think that is our answer.'

'That's no answer,' she boomed. 'I came here for you to fix his teeth in his head. Are you going to do it or not?'

By this time Sandra was beginning to be affected by the mounting tension of the situation. Her blank expression was now replaced by one of fear as she saw Mrs Hitchcock becoming redder by the minute. She was clearly terrified of Mrs Hitchcock which was not surprising; I was very wary of her myself and conscious of the fact that I was annoying her, but I wasn't going to let her come into my surgery and dictate what treatment I should provide especially when it was contrary to my clinical judgment. I paused for a moment then began to speak in a tone of voice which I hoped would sound authoritative.

'I think that you and Mr Hitchcock had better talk it over together. Personally, I take Mr Hitchcock's view that, in the circumstances, the best course of action is to do nothing. I'm not prepared to reline the dentures anyway because I don't think that is the answer. It's new dentures or nothing; the choice is yours.'

I took the bowl containing Mr Hitchcock's dentures and offered it to him. He took out the contents and slipped them into his mouth with practised ease.

Mrs Hitchcock was white with temper, mainly I think because I had taken the side of her husband. She jumped to her feet and looked so menacing that Sandra fled from the room.

'I have never heard anything so ridiculous' she exploded. 'We come in here with a simple enough request, which any dentist worthy of the name would be able to carry out without any fuss or argument, but not you. Oh, no. You have to make things complicated, then you have the nerve to stick up for him. You've played right into his hands, haven't you? He didn't want to come here in the first place and you've as good as given him your blessing to carry on driving me crazy with his loose teeth. I can't stand it any more. Come on, Harold, get out of that chair. There's going to be a bloody row when we get home.'

Mrs Hitchcock had made so much noise that Spencer came along to see what was going on.

'The Hitchcocks ,was it?' he smirked.

'Yes, do you know them?'

'Oh, yes, very well. Let me guess – Mrs Hitchcock's being driven mad by her husband's loose and clicking dentures? Wants a new lining fitted to give them more grip on to the gums, whilst he thinks they are fine? They will be back again in about six months to try again, which is something for you to look forward to. I've seen them at least three times in the last two years. Mrs H. didn't get anywhere with me. so she thought she'd give you a try. How is Sandra getting on?'

'Mrs Hitchcock scared the living daylights out of her. I think she's in the office. I'd better go and find her.'

CHAPTER THIRTEEN

'Has she gone?' were Sandra's first words.

'Yes, she's gone. Our next patient is here. Her name is Mrs Gunn. She isn't like Mrs Hitchcock, you'll be all right with her. Go and fetch her from the waiting room.'

Mrs Gunn was more than a little eccentric and somewhat highly strung, but generally quite pleasant. She tended to over-react to most situations and the first few minutes of each appointment were usually spent telling me how much pain she had suffered after the last filling I had done for her. However, she kept returning for more treatment, so I had come to accept her moans as a matter of course.

'This is Sandra, Mrs Gunn. It's her first day with me today.'

'I don't think I could do the job, Sandra. You must be very brave to take it on what with all that blood and mess and looking into people's smelly mouths all day. Ugh, I don't envy you one little bit.'

'It's not too bad, Mrs Gunn,' I returned quickly, thinking that this was not what I wanted Sandra to be hearing. 'Sandra is doing very well, and she'll soon get used to it. Today,' I continued for Sandra's benefit, 'we're going to do the last of Mrs Gunn's fillings and then we're going to take some impressions for a new partial denture.'

I saw Sandra's face drop once again at the mention of a denture. 'Can we have a denture bowl for Mrs Gunn, please? No, not that one. Take one from the cupboard.'

Sandra put down the bowl that had contained Mr Hitchcock's dentures and found a clean one, which she offered to Mrs Gunn with a look of utter distaste. She held it in front of Mrs Gunn for a brief moment with her eyes tightly closed, then snatched it away so quickly that Mrs Gunn missed it as she tried to place her denture in it. The pink plastic plate landed on her lap. Luckily it didn't fall on the floor.

'Sorry,' stammered Sandra, upset because she knew she was making a mess of things.

I took the bowl from Sandra. I knew there was no way she would touch Mrs Gunn's denture with her hands so I picked it up myself and, after rinsing it under the tap, I placed it safely in the bowl.

Anxious to move on I turned to Sandra and said, 'we'll do Mrs Gunn's filling now, so if you pass me a syringe I'll numb her tooth before we start.'

Sandra, however, didn't move. She just stared back at me, her face contorted with pain and anguish. 'A syringe please, Sandra.' I repeated. 'In the top drawer, just to your right.' Still she made no attempt to fulfil my request. Rather than ask her again I went to the drawer and took out a syringe myself. As I unsheathed the needle I saw Sandra gasp for breath and I realised at that moment that in addition to all her other phobias she also had a dread of needles. She turned deathly white and I saw her reel backwards, steadying herself against the instrument cabinet. I was sure she was going to fall down and I was about to run over to catch her. Somehow, however, she managed to regain some composure and, when I was reasonably sure she would remain on her feet, I administered the injection. She was still hanging onto the cabinet for support and had turned her face towards the wall so that she would not have to witness what to her was a horrifying spectacle.

By the time I had finished drilling the tooth, Sandra had recovered sufficiently to take some interest in the placing of the filling.

'We need to line the cavity before we fill it,' I explained to Sandra. 'Mix together this powder and this liquid to a stiff paste.' I thought that this would be simple enough for her to perform and hoped that it might provide a little interest and boost her confidence. Unfortunately the screw cap on the bottle of liquid was too tight for her to remove, but at least the effort of trying to unscrew it brought back some colour to her cheeks. In the end she realised she was not going to be able to manage it, admitted defeat and handed the bottle to me.

I loosened the cap and gave the bottle of powder back to her. Sadly, the events of the morning had worked Sandra into such a state of nerves that she was all fingers and thumbs. After removing the cap she accidentally dropped the jar, spilling white flour-like powder over herself, the worktop, the floor and into a half open drawer containing dental instruments.

'Oh no,' she screamed. 'I'm useless. I can't do anything.'

'Don't worry,' I said calmly, realising that the poor girl was very close to tears. 'We'll clean it up later.'

'I'm always dropping things,' added Mrs Gunn reassuringly, sensing Sandra's distress.

'Well, you expect to at your age,' Sandra retorted fiercely, not really intending the remark to be as offensive as it sounded. She was clearly very unhappy and was not going to be consoled easily.

'If you like, you can just watch,' I said to her, 'until you feel a bit more confident.'

I completed the filling of Mrs Gunn's tooth without further help or hindrance from Sandra, who stood looking sullenly on from a respectable distance.

'Now we have finished all your fillings, Mrs Gunn, we can get started on making you a new partial denture.'

'Yes, Mr Derwent, I shall be so glad to get a new one. This one has been quite good but I feel that the time has come now for something better. I was talking to a friend about it and she told me that there are lots of different types of denture. Is that true?'

'Yes, it is. There are many variations in design, it is a question of selecting the most suitable type for each case and then, of course, there are a number of different materials we can choose from.'

'What is the very best type to have? I don't like wearing a denture but, since I have no choice, I would like to think I am wearing the very best available.'

'I think in your case a metal skeleton denture would be most suitable.'

'Oh, Mr Derwent, that sounds awful. What on earth is a skeleton denture?'

'Well, instead of having a big plate that takes up a lot of room in your mouth, a skeleton denture has just thin bars so there is much less of it. In order to be strong enough though it has to be made of metal. The plastic material that your existing denture is made of wouldn't be strong enough for this sort of design.'

'I like the idea of it being less bulky but what sort of metal would you use. It isn't going to be pink coloured is it? So it won't look very good.'

'It's only the framework that would be metal and that isn't going to show very much. The teeth themselves would match your own.'

'But people might catch a glimpse of it if I open my mouth wide. Would it be stainless steel or that sort of colour?'

'Yes, probably, though it would be chrome-cobalt rather than stainless steel, but the colour is much the same.'

'I don't think I would like that, Mr Derwent. Isn't there anything else you could use that would look better?'

'It could be gold, though it would be very expensive. The yellow colour of gold blends in much better than a silver metal, and if it did show a bit people might just think you had gold fillings.'

'Now I do like the sound of that, Mr Derwent. Oh yes. That must be the very best possible denture one could have.'

'It certainly would, Mrs Gunn, but as I said it would be awfully expensive.'

'I don't care about that. I said I wanted the very best and I don't mind how much it costs.'

'Very well, Mrs Gunn, a gold denture it is then. We'll take some impressions and get started on it right away.'

After Mrs Gunn had left Sandra began to show some interest. 'Will it be very expensive to make a denture out of gold?' she asked in a tone of voice, which implied that she thought the whole idea was ridiculous.

'I would imagine so,' I replied thoughtfully. 'I've never actually made one before so I don't know exactly, but it will probably cost at least three or four times more than an ordinary metal denture. Still, you heard what Mrs Gunn said; she wants the best and doesn't mind paying for it. There are a lot of people in this area who are very wealthy.'

'It must be wonderful to be so rich that you don't have to worry about how expensive things are,' said Sandra wistfully. 'She didn't even want to know the actual price.'

'No, she didn't. She probably is very well off, though she doesn't look it particularly, does she? Her clothes aren't anything special, but you can't necessarily go by that. Some very rich people walk around looking like tramps. Anyway, if she had been concerned about the price she would have asked me to give her a quote for it.'

For a few moments Sandra had seemed a little more relaxed as we discussed Mrs Gunn's wealth and we managed to clean up the spilt powder without much trouble. I hoped that nothing else would happen to upset her.

Suddenly Spencer appeared at the door. He always arranged his appointments so that he had a few minutes breathing space between patients. Good for helping to keep the blood pressure under control but not so good for someone like me who was well aware that when you weren't actually treating a patient you weren't making any money. My overdraft was not showing any signs of coming down – in fact quite the reverse – because however hard I tried to avoid it, my expenditure always seemed to exceed my income.

'How are you getting on with Mrs Gunn?' he began.

'Pretty well. She's only decided to have a gold denture.'

'What?' gasped Spencer his facing lighting up. 'How splendid. How much have you quoted her for it?'

Although Spencer was not disposed to working hard himself to earn lots of money, he was as keen as anyone to see his bank balance increase, especially when it didn't require any effort from himself. When I succeeded in selling expensive dentistry, as my principal he naturally benefited from it and he was not ungrateful.

'I haven't. She said she didn't care about the cost, just wanted the best.'

'Good grief, Justin, that's marvellous. I had no idea the Gunns were that well-off; they don't drive an expensive car. I suppose some people don't believe in spending lots of money on cars, but we don't mind that as long as they are prepared to spend it on their teeth. I obviously should have taken them on to my books. You ought to phone the laboratory and get some idea what their bill will be, then we can work out a price. I always think that it is best to submit accounts in guineas to private patients. It sounds more professional.'

'Guineas? I didn't think anyone used guineas these days.'

'They do in professional circles. My solicitor always sends his bills in guineas.'

I got the feeling that Spencer was already planning how he intended to spend his share of the profit. When he left to return to his surgery he was still smiling all over his face and muttering that one should never prejudge how much people are able and willing to spend on their teeth.

CHAPTER FOURTEEN

I was aware that I was running late. After only a short time in general practice I had come to realise that when carrying out dentistry it was very common for things to take longer than had been allowed for. Sometimes it was because the actual operation proved more difficult than expected and sometimes it was because patients asked questions or insisted on talking about something. When I ran late, then inevitably, the next patient was kept waiting. Most of them didn't mind too much, but some objected very strongly. My next patient was Major Hetherington-Smythe and he was a stickler for punctuality.

I was very concerned that he would be in the waiting room complaining bitterly to anyone else who happened to be with him. On this occasion, however, he had become so upset about being kept waiting ten minutes that he came upstairs and he was, at that moment, venting his anger on poor Beryl.

I guessed what had happened when I heard his raised voice and so I went to meet him, hoping that I might be able to pacify him. I thought there was no point in sending Sandra to do the job as she would not be capable of facing up to him.

'I am so dreadfully sorry, Major,' I grovelled. 'I was unavoidably detained with the last patient and, on this occasion, I just couldn't help running late. I appreciate that you don't like being kept waiting and I would have avoided it if at all possible. I promise it won't happen again.' I really felt like saying that I had only kept him waiting ten minutes, for heaven's sake, that it was well nigh impossible to keep absolutely to time in a job like this and that if he wanted to be sure of being seen on time he should arrange to come to the first appointment in the morning, not towards the end of the session. The Major refused, however, to make any appointments before eleven o'clock in the morning.

'Damn poor show, Derwent,' he barked. 'Keeping me waiting suggests that you think your time's more precious than mine. Well, let me tell you, it isn't. If we make an appointment for eleven o'clock I expect to be seen at eleven o'clock, not five past, not ten past; eleven o'clock.'

I could feel my hackles beginning to rise at what I considered to be total unreasonableness on his part, but I kept calm.

'I accept what you are saying, Major, but I can do no more than apologise profusely. Would you like to come through to the surgery now so that I can get on with your treatment? Whilst we are standing here talking I am getting later still, so the next patient is going to be kept waiting even longer. That wouldn't be fair to them, would it?'

'Now look here, Derwent, I hope you aren't going to hurry my treatment in an attempt to catch up. I was booked in for an hour and I expect to get an hour.'

'You are here to have three teeth extracted, Major. I allowed an hour so that I would have plenty of time. It doesn't normally take an hour to extract three teeth, and I hope it won't in your case. I can take an hour over it if you wish, but surely you would rather get it over and done with as quickly as possible.'

Put like that he could hardly argue but I was rapidly coming to the conclusion that Major Hetherington-Smythe simply enjoyed arguing and being difficult.

'I'm telling you that I want a proper job done. I don't expect to feel any pain and I don't want to feel that you rushed the job. Now let's get on with it, but I can tell you I'm not looking forward to this one little bit.'

'It will be fine, Major. The teeth are actually quite loose, so it shouldn't be difficult to extract them.'

'It's getting them numb that I'm worried about. Last dentist I went to had a devil of a job with anything in the lower jaw. Told me I must have an extra nerve in my neck or some such thing. Anyway he could never numb them properly. Felt everything he did every time.'

'I've got some new very strong anaesthetic which I use in difficult cases like yours. It should do the trick without any problem at all.'

I got the Major seated in the dental chair and Sandra, with a little prompting from me, proceeded to hang a bib round his neck.

'I say, steady on. Not so tight, you're not supposed to strangle me with it you know,' snapped the Major. Poor Sandra took it as a bitter attack and shrank away looking completely demoralised. As she saw me take out a syringe to administer the anaesthetic, she rapidly turned her head away.

'Open as wide as you can, please Major... Wider please... Really wide.'

'Don't be ridiculous, man, I'm at full stretch now. What the hell do you expect? I haven't got a mouth like a hippopotamus you know.'

I was sure that he was making only a half-hearted attempt to open his mouth, but there was no point in arguing with someone like Major Hetherington-Smythe. If he didn't open his mouth wide it made it more difficult for me to gauge where to place the needle and it occurred to me that this might be why previous dentists had found it difficult to get him numb. If the anaesthetic solution was not injected in exactly the right place then it wouldn't work properly. Working under difficult circumstances, I chose the spot to insert the needle. As soon as it touched his gum, the Major let out an ear-splitting shriek and dragged my hand and the syringe, away from his mouth.

'Christ Almighty. What the bloody hell are you trying to do to me? That was excruciating. Surely it shouldn't hurt as much as that. Do you know what you are doing?'

'I can assure you I do, Major. It would hurt less if you kept still and I must warn you about grabbing hold of my hand whilst I'm holding a needle. It could be dangerous.'

'Well, what the hell do you expect? That was more than flesh and blood can stand. Can't you rub something on the gum to deaden it a bit before you stick the damn needle in?'

' Okay. Let's try this,' I said, trying not to appear too concerned about the fact that so far I wasn't scoring too highly with him. I rubbed some topical anaesthetic cream on to the area where I was trying to insert the needle. It was right at the back of the mouth and I waited a few moments before I received the reaction I was expecting.

A look of anguish started to spread across the Major's face. Suddenly he clutched at his throat. 'Bloody hell,' he spluttered. 'I'm choking. My throat's closing up. I can't swallow, I can't breathe.'

'Relax, Major,' I said softly and reassuringly without a trace of anxiety. 'You aren't choking – it's just that the cream is numbing your throat and some people find it a bit unpleasant. That is why I tend not to use it if it can be avoided, but you needed something to make the injection less painful so we had to give it a try. The feeling will wear off quite quickly and I can assure you that you won't choke.'

The Major didn't look convinced. His already ruddy features were becoming more and more colourful by the second. He was retching and coughing and his eyes were bulging dramatically behind his horn-rimmed spectacles.

'Just lie back and take some deep breaths,' I said, gently pushing him back into the chair. I handed him a glass. 'Take some sips of water.'

He did as I said and began to calm down a little. 'Now,' I said, 'we need to get the injection in before the numbness from the paste wears off.'

I think the exertion from coughing, spluttering and gasping for breath had exhausted him for the moment and I was able to administer the injection with no more than a few squirms, groans and some flapping of the arms by way of protest. I prayed that I had managed to hit the right spot and that the anaesthetic would take quickly and profoundly, though under the circumstances it would be a minor miracle if it happened.

'Something's happening,' announced the Major. 'My lip's going dead. Look, I can bite it quite hard and I don't feel it.'

'I wouldn't do that if I were you. When it comes round you will have a very sore lip and no doubt you will swear that I caused it.'

He didn't answer; he just sat there staring into space. His breathing was rapid and shallow and there was an air of inevitability about his expression. Sandra who had witnessed all this without a single word looked terrified. The pallor of her skin was in complete contrast to the scarlet complexion of the patient.

'Can't we get on with it, Derwent?'

'I want to be sure you are numb. I'll test it with this sharp probe.' I pushed the sharp tip into his gum. He didn't flinch.

'There, you didn't feel that, did you?'

'Feel what? Do it again.'

Once again I pressed the sharp tip of the probe into his gum. I said, 'I think it is fairly clear that you can't feel anything. Is that right?'

'Looks that way,' he conceded.

'Very well then, we'll have those teeth out in no time. Will you pass me the forceps please, Sandra?'

I should have known better than to ask her. I suppose I had been so concerned with trying to deal with the Major that I had temporarily forgotten about her hang-ups. I was very quickly reminded.

'No, no, I can't bear the sight of blood. I can't stay here if there is going to be blood.'

She looked as if she was about to burst into tears once again and I could see that there was no point in trying to coax her or comfort her.

'All right, Sandra. Go and see if Beryl is free, and ask her to come in and help me.'

Sandra immediately latched on to the opportunity to get out of the room and was gone like a shot. Luckily Beryl was able to come and assist so I set about relieving the Major of his troublesome teeth.

'Thanks for coming to help, Beryl. Will you just steady the Major's head?'

Beryl knew exactly what to do and positioned herself behind the chair with her hands gently but firmly on each side of his head to help prevent it from moving around caused either by his struggles to escape, or by my struggles to extract the teeth.

I tried to position the forceps on one of the doomed teeth but it was so loose I had to stabilise it with a finger in order to close the beaks of the instrument around it. I tightened my grip.

'Jesus Christ,' screamed the Major. 'Stop, stop.' I released my grip on the tooth. 'That's agonisingly painful,' he moaned, his face contorted. 'I need more jungle juice.'

'It seemed numb enough when I tested it just now.' I picked up the probe and tested the gum around the tooth once again. The Major obviously felt nothing, so I gave the tooth a smart tap with the handle of my mouth mirror. 'Is it tender when I do that?'

'Well no, but it hurt like hell when you tried to pull it out.'

'I didn't actually get to the point of trying to pull it. I had hardly taken hold of it with the forceps when you screamed.'

I was convinced that the tooth was numb and to prove the point, whilst I was talking and pretending to be checking for numbness, I took hold of the tooth with my finger and thumb and gave it a quick twist. A look of amazement came over the Major's face as I held the tooth up for him to see.

'It's out,' I declared triumphantly.

'What? It's out?'

'You can see it is, Major. You didn't feel anything at all did you?'

'I think I felt something but it wasn't as bad as the first time you tried. I suppose what happened was that you loosened it with the pliers, which was the painful bit, and then you were able to pluck it out with your fingers.'

There seemed little point in telling him that I didn't really get hold of it with the forceps and that the only actual extraction force I applied was with my fingers. The main thing was that the tooth was out; one down and two more to go. Unfortunately, the other two, although mobile, were somewhat tighter and not loose enough for me to extract with my fingers.

'Okay. Let's try the next one. This shouldn't be any trouble either.'

As soon as I closed the forceps on to it he let out a piercing cry, which could probably have been heard throughout Luccombury.

'Bloody hell.' His hands shot up to his face and he wrenched my hand away from his mouth. 'Christ, Derwent, you certainly know how to inflict pain. I told you I need more jungle juice.'

'I can't understand it, Major. The whole of that side of your jaw seems to be completely numb. It shouldn't be hurting like that.'

'You're damn right it shouldn't. I'm beginning to think you have no idea what you are doing. Have you taken any teeth out before, or am I your first victim?'

'I can assure you I have taken out many teeth. I have tested your gum to check that the anaesthetic has worked and there is no doubt that it has taken effect. What you are feeling is simply pressure and there is no way to avoid that. If you can't stand it, if it really is too painful for you to tolerate because you have a low pain threshold, then the only way round it is to send you to the hospital and they will put you to sleep to do the job.'

'Low pain threshold? What the bloody hell are you talking about? I was hit twice by enemy fire during the war. One of the chaps took a piece of shrapnel from my shoulder out in the field. Like to see you youngsters face what we had to go through, and you try to tell me I have a low pain threshold. I find that bloody insulting.'

Up to a point, it was intended to be. I had a strong suspicion he would be the type to be proud of his war record. Maybe his pride was justified, I don't know. I was simply attempting to use the fact that, in the light of his rank and military history, he would not want to appear less than highly courageous whatever the situation.

I continued. 'Well, Major, as I see it, we have to make a decision. I can give you some more anaesthetic, but I don't think it will make a lot of difference because I am sure that you are quite numb. I think you must accept that if I carry on and extract these teeth it will be uncomfortable. If you think you can stand it then fine and I can assure you it will all be over and done with very quickly; in a matter of seconds in fact. On the other hand, if you don't feel you can face it we will abandon the attempt and I will write a letter of referral to the hospital, though it could take several weeks before you get an appointment.'

The Major looked as if he had been trapped in a corner. 'Oh bloody well get on with it, Derwent. No-one tells me I've got a low pain threshold.'

'Very well, Major as long as you are sure.'

I picked up the forceps again and Beryl renewed her hold of the Major's head. It took less than a minute to remove the other two teeth. It would have taken less had it not been for the screams, the swearing and the wriggling. Fortunately there were no other patients in the waiting room to hear what was going on.

'Thank God that's over,' the Major exclaimed. 'That was bloody agony, Derwent, bloody agony.'

'Well, at least the teeth are out now and won't give you any further trouble. Now I want you to listen carefully to what I am going to say. It is extremely important that you follow these instructions. I have placed a gauze pad in your mouth, I want you to keep biting hard on it for half an hour, then you can remove it and throw it away. You must try to avoid eating on that side for a few days and don't under any circumstances be tempted to rinse your mouth today as you will disturb the blood clot and start the sockets bleeding again. Is that quite clear?'

'Perfectly, Derwent. You don't need to treat me like a fool. I have had teeth out before you know.'

'Well just to be sure, I will give you these written instructions.'

'I've told you, I don't need them. What I need is a large Scotch, not some bloody instructions.'

I was going to tell him about the danger of drinking alcohol after a tooth extraction and that I didn't advise it, then decided I wouldn't bother.

CHAPTER FIFTEEN

After the Major had left, I went back into the office where Sandra was sitting staring out of the window looking as if she had all the troubles of the world on her shoulders.

'Don't worry,' I said to her. 'You will get used to it in time. It hasn't been an easy morning for you so far but the last two patients of the morning are just for check-ups and X-rays so that shouldn't be too bad. Let me teach you a little bit about the way we fill in the record cards, as we have about ten minutes before Mr and Mrs Blenkinsopp are due.'

Sandra seemed to cheer up a little and showed genuine interest in learning how to chart teeth. In fact, she learnt quite quickly and with a little guidance was able to fill in the little boxes on the record cards as I called out the cavities.

Mrs Blenkinsopp's teeth were quite good but Mr Blenkinsopp was a dentist's nightmare. He was a habitual mint eater having given up smoking about three years ago, and he always put lots of sugar into the many cups of tea and coffee he consumed every day. He admitted that he had an uncontrollable liking for anything sweet and, to make matters worse, he cleaned his teeth only occasionally and didn't make a very good job of it either. He was extremely prone to getting cavities in his teeth. He and his wife came every six months for their check-ups, as regular as clockwork. Every time, Mr Blenkinsopp needed lots of filling and several appointments had to be made for him. By the time the course of treatment was completed it was almost time for his next check-up. Fillings never seemed to last very long in his mouth and either fell out or had to be replaced because there was more decay at the margins. It was like painting the Forth Bridge, though it didn't seem to worry him too much.

'How many fillings is it this time then, Mr Derwent?' As if he were trying to set up an all time record for producing the highest number of cavities in six months. 'Fifteen, is it? That's not as many as last time.'

'Well we haven't taken X-rays yet. We might find some more. Come this way.'

I led him through to the office and sat him in the chair alongside the huge black X-ray machine. It seemed ancient compared with the streamlined modern machines we had at dental school. Spencer was convinced that it was every bit as good as the new machines on the market; in fact he claimed it was superior in many respects.

I wasn't so sure. I was particularly concerned that it made a rather strange crackling sound every time you took an X-ray and there was no doubt that the noise was getting worse. The noise was there again when I X-rayed Mr Blenkinsopp's teeth; it didn't sound right at all to me.

I spoke to Spencer about it after the Blenkinsopps had left, but he dismissed my concerns immediately.

'It's absolutely nothing to worry about. Old X-ray machines are like old cars; they're bound to be a bit noisy compared with their more modern counterparts, but that doesn't mean there is anything wrong. I tell you Justin, this old machine will still be going strong in twenty years' time.'

'Has it always crackled like that?'

He looked somewhat vague. 'Well, yes, I think so. I don't know, really. I suppose if I'm honest it makes a bit more noise than it used to, but that's only to be expected. I can assure you it is perfectly all right. You have only to look at the results we get from it to see that it is in perfect working order.'

'Well, that's just the point, Spencer. Some of the X-ray pictures I've taken recently weren't that clear; they were very faint and not of much diagnostic value.'

'You probably didn't angle the beam properly, or maybe the chemicals in the developer need changing. All the X-ray pictures I've taken have been perfect.'

'Well, that's my next point,' I continued. 'I don't think we change the chemicals often enough. The developer was the colour of cold tea when I looked at it last week, and mighty strong tea at that. We ought to be changing it every two weeks to be sure that we are getting the best possible results. Once it has darkened beyond a pale straw colour it isn't much good any more.'

'Rubbish,' Spencer interjected. 'The manufacturers of the stuff want you to change it frequently because they sell more that way. It lasts much longer than they say it does; it certainly isn't necessary to change it as often as every two weeks. Every two months is more like it.' With that he flounced out before I had time to say anything else.

Sandra didn't say much more to me before she left to go home for lunch. She seemed very relieved to have come to the end of the morning and could hardly get out quickly enough. I hoped that there had been parts of the morning that she had found interesting and that she realised it would take some time before she got used to the job. Whilst I didn't think she was ideally suited to it, I was prepared to be patient with her and try to help her overcome her phobias. I knew though that it wouldn't be easy and that it might be some time before I could rely upon her to give me the sort of help a dentist expects from his nurse.

After lunch I got back to the surgery in good time to prepare for the first patient of the afternoon. I hoped that Sandra would also be early so that I could explain to her what I would be doing and give her a few instructions on how she could best assist me. The patient was a delightful little six-year-old girl who needed a small filling. I had treated her before and she was an excellent patient. She had no fear of dentists, didn't need injections and just sat there quietly with her mouth wide open enabling me to carry out the treatment without any difficulty. I thought this would be ideal for Sandra. No needles, no blood, no dentures; it should launch her into the afternoon in the best possible way.

The patient was due at two o'clock and arrived with her mother exactly on time. Sandra had not arrived at five past so I thought I ought to carry on without her as I hated keeping patients waiting if I could avoid it. The treatment went according to plan and the tooth was drilled and the filling placed by twenty-five past, even though I had no chair side assistance.

Spencer popped his head round my door. He was looking slightly dishevelled and a bit bleary eyed having just got up from his customary post-prandial nap. 'Has Sandra not turned up yet?' he asked.

'No, I have no idea where she can be. I am sure she knows we start back at two in the afternoon, though I didn't manage to speak to her before she left for lunch.'

'I'm going to the bank in a moment. I go past where she lives so I'll call in and see if she's all right.'

'Fine, thanks, Spencer.'

It was about three quarters of an hour later when he came back, and he didn't look particularly pleased. I wasn't terribly pleased either because I was having to perform the role of dental nurse as well as dentist, which wasn't always easy. There were times when it was necessary to have another pair of hands available to help, even if they weren't very skilled hands. Beryl had been on the telephone for the whole of the time that Spencer was away. Heaven knows who she had been talking to all that time, but it meant that I had been forced to work completely unaided.

He came straight up to my surgery. 'You swine,' he exclaimed, 'you rotten swine. What the hell did you do to her? The poor girl's a quivering wreck. She's sitting at home in floods of tears, utterly inconsolable. She cannot face coming back to work for you. That's it, she's quit. You've destroyed her completely in just one morning. I think you've driven her to a nervous breakdown. How the hell you managed it in just one morning I shall never know, but you have. God knows, Justin, you are going to have to be a bit more tolerant and understanding with your nurses. You can't afford to be a complete and utter bastard to them, or you'll never get anyone to come and work for you.'

'Oh come on, Spencer,' I protested. 'I didn't do anything to her, she just wasn't cut out for the job. Anyway, more to the point, what am I going to do for a nurse now? I can't manage on my own.'

Spencer looked worried. 'I'll find you someone else. In the meantime I'll try and get Daphne to help you out. She has worked with me in the surgery from time to time so she has a fair idea what it's all about. She hasn't done much for a few years now so she is bound to be a bit rusty but I'm sure she will be quite useful to you. She isn't in at the moment and I'm not sure what time she'll be back, but if you try to manage as best you can for the time being I'll speak to her as soon as she gets in. You can also share Beryl with me. She'll give you a hand this afternoon. I'm not all that busy so she should be available to help you.'

'But she can't help me and you, and answer the telephone and the doorbell as well.'

'Don't worry, Justin, it will be fine. You'll get through somehow. It's amazing how one seems to be able to cope in difficult circumstances when one has to.' And with that he breezed out of my surgery leaving me feeling slightly annoyed. Sandra had obviously been entirely the wrong choice. Spencer should have known that she would never be any good as a dental nurse. Either he hadn't bothered to interview her properly to assess her suitability for the job or his desperation to fill the post overrode common sense. I was annoyed that he hadn't taken more care to find someone who at least didn't have a total aversion to dentures, blood and needles especially as he refused to let me play any part in the selection process. I was also annoyed that he had now landed me in the situation of not having anyone to help me in the surgery. He was perfectly content to potter along at a leisurely pace allowing loads of time for each patient, but I had a large overdraft and needed to earn money to pay it off. In order to do that I needed to work hard and efficiently and it wasn't going to be easy to do that without a nurse to help me. Anyway, there wasn't much I could do about it except hope that Daphne would prove useful in the meantime and that Spencer would quickly find me another nurse, only this time, she would be someone more suited to the job.

I managed to get through the rest of the afternoon without too much difficulty because Beryl spent quite a lot of time helping me, more, in fact, than she spent with Spencer. I got the feeling that Spencer, sensing that I was upset at being left without a nurse, decided that he would have to let Beryl work with me as much as possible even though he might himself suffer some inconvenience as a result.

I was just finishing a filling on who I thought was my last patient of the afternoon when the telephone rang. Beryl answered it and it was Major Hetherington-Smythe on the other end, in quite a state of hysteria because apparently he was still bleeding profusely from the extractions I had performed for him that morning. I instructed Beryl to tell him to come to the surgery straight away.

Beryl had hardly put down the phone when the doorbell rang and there he was.

'He must have been jet propelled,' I said to her as she went escort him from the waiting room. At least I wouldn't have to hang around waiting for him to arrive as so often happens when you ask patients to come straight round. When they say they will be with you within ten minutes it is invariably twenty or more before they turn up.

The Major mounted the stairs three steps at a time and burst into my surgery.

'You've butchered me, Derwent. Still bleeding like a stuck pig. Tried everything to stop it. I've rinsed it with salt water, TCP, glycerin and thymol, whisky; got through the best part of a bottle of Scotch since lunchtime but I can't stop the damn thing bleeding. I reckon you hit a blood vessel or something.'

'I didn't hit anything, Major. They were perfectly straightforward extractions. Do you remember the instructions I gave you this morning?'

'Instructions? What instructions? You didn't give me any. What could you have told me that I didn't already know anyway? There wasn't much to say, was there? What the hell could I do more than I have already done to stop it bleeding? The reason the damn thing won't stop in this case is perfectly obvious; you bloody well butchered me. The way you pulled and tugged at me you have probably torn the gums to ribbons. I suppose you'll have to sew me up now?'

I indicated to him to sit in the dental chair. 'I'm afraid the reason the bleeding hasn't stopped is down to you.'

'What the hell are you talking about? That just about takes the biscuit. You make a bloody mess of things and then try to blame it on me. That's just about typical of you youngsters. You've made a hash of this one, Derwent. I'd respect you more if you owned up to it but to try and blame me for it, that's despicable.'

'Major, I told you this morning not to rinse your mouth today because this would wash away the blood clot and keep it bleeding, and what did you do? You went home and rinsed with everything you could lay your hands on. It's no wonder you're still bleeding.'

'Rubbish. First of all I don't remember you telling me not to rinse, and in any case I can't believe that it would do any harm. I think you're just making excuses because you know damn well you've butchered me. Just get me sewn up and I'll be on my way. I've spent enough time in this damn hell hole today.'

I cleaned out his mouth with some gauze and then rolled up another piece to form a pad. I placed it on top of the extraction sockets and instructed him to bite hard on it.

'Now I want you to sit there for half an hour, keeping firm biting pressure on that gauze pad the whole time.'

The major tried to protest through clenched jaws. 'What about stitching it up...' he began, but I stopped him.

'Don't try to talk. Say nothing, do nothing, just sit there in silence for half an hour. Here is a magazine to read. I will come back when your time's up.'

I went out into the office and took the opportunity to do some paper work. After exactly half an hour I went back and removed the gauze from the Major's mouth. 'There you are, Major, the bleeding has stopped. Now go home and do not under any circumstances do anything which might disturb the blood clot, which means do not rinse your mouth for the next twenty four hours. Have you got that?'

'What about stitching it?'

'Not necessary. It will be fine as long as you do as I say. No rinsing. Is that perfectly clear?'

'I thought rinsing it would help keep it free of infection and make it heal up quicker.'

'You mustn't rinse for twenty-four hours. Is that absolutely clear? I suggest you come and let me have another look at you tomorrow afternoon. Can you manage that?'

'Yes if you consider it to be necessary, but I still think you ought to stitch the gums.'

'Come about four o'clock then, Major, and take it easy this evening. Nothing too strenuous and no rinsing, and go easy on the Scotch.'

CHAPTER SIXTEEN

It was a cold damp evening as I pushed open the creaking old gate and made my way with some trepidation towards Dr MacKean's surgery door. A dim light above the door lit up the path and enabled me to negotiate a route around the overgrown vegetation. The brass sign on the wall was badly in need of metal polish, though there was no doubt that it had received its fair share of polish in the past because large areas of brass had been rubbed away. This made it difficult to read the name but, according to Spencer, Dr Mackean had been around for many many years, everybody knew him, and so I suppose the sign was no longer of great importance. The brass door handle was similarly tarnished and the door itself was in need of repainting. The doorframe was so rotten it looked as if it might come away from the wall if someone shut the door too hard.

My heart was pounding as I stepped into the small, gloomy waiting room. It was pretty unwelcoming with once cream paint on the walls, which had long since faded to a dirty yellow, green linoleum on the floor, and a number of old leather seated oak dining chairs in neat rows against every bit of available wall space.

There was a strange smell of mustiness combined with antiseptic, and for some reason my first reaction was that it was like visiting the premises of a back street abortionist – not that I had ever actually been to an abortionist's premises – but I felt sure that this was what it would be like.

I hated the idea of a medical examination and for this reason I had been apprehensive when I arrived. Now, having seen Dr MacKean's waiting room, I began to feel extremely nervous.

I kept telling myself to take some deep breaths and try to calm down. After all, it was only an insurance medical and Spencer said there wouldn't be any problem with Dr Mackean.

The waiting room was completely empty and in fact there didn't seem to be anyone in the house at all. I listened carefully but I couldn't hear any signs of movement or voices. I didn't quite know what to do so I just stood staring at a faded old watercolour painting on the wall. Dr MacKean had asked me to attend at seven o'clock by which time he would have finished his evening surgery. It was five to seven by my watch so I decided to wait a bit longer before trying to find someone.

I walked round the waiting room looking at the other pictures on the wall. They were all of a similar age and had probably adorned the walls since ever since Dr MacKean had set up practice there. I wondered how many patients had looked at them over the years. Spencer's waiting room wasn't exactly spick and span but compared with this it was luxurious. I realised, however, that Dr MacKean had probably been in practice much longer than Spencer. From what I had heard, it sounded as though Dr MacKean was not far from retirement. What would Spencer's waiting room look like when he reached that stage?

At a couple of minutes past seven, the door on the opposite wall to where I had entered suddenly opened and a white-haired gentleman appeared. He was heavily built with pronounced jowls and must have been well into his sixties. He wore gold half-moon glasses and walked with a slight stoop.

'Hello, you must be Justin. Balfour MacKean at your service. Do come through to the surgery.' We shook hands and I followed him through.

The surgery had the same grubby paint on the walls and the same worn green linoleum on the floor. Against one wall was an ancient, perhaps antique, leather examination couch. There were several holes in it where the padding was sticking out and folded neatly at one end was a tartan blanket. Dr MacKean's desk was set diagonally across one corner of the room and was absolutely weighted down with papers and patients' record cards scattered haphazardly in untidy heaps over the entire desktop.

It was definitely the surgery of an old doctor and although completely lacking in any sort of refinement, it had a certain air of informality and, in a strange way, a cosiness about it, which made it seem less daunting. I think the crowning glory was the bare electric light bulb, which hung from the centre of the ceiling. In spite of the fact that the light from the bulb was not diminished or impeded by the presence of a shade, the accumulation of dust and low wattage of the bulb ensured that the room was very dimly lit.

'Do take a seat, Justin,' Dr MacKean began. 'Spencer phoned me and told me who you were. He asked me to treat you gently. I understand you haven't been in general practice very long?'

'That's right. I've only just left university, and this is my first job.'

'How are you getting on? Do you like it?'

'Yes, thank you. I'm settling in. I get on well with Spencer and I like working with him.'

'He's got a very good sense of humour though I know his father better. He and I play golf together sometimes.'

'I'm sorry to keep you here so late, Dr MacKean.'

'That's all right. I often stay here until nine or ten o'clock. I try to catch up with my paperwork though, as you can see, I still have a long way to go. Just look at this lot,' pointing to the jumble on his desk. 'I don't think I shall ever be up to date. If I'm honest about it, I'm as happy here as I am at home. I'm my own boss here and I don't have to put up with my wife nagging me. In any case, you need plenty of time for an insurance medical so I always do them after I have finished with all my other patients.'

I was hoping that it would all be over in a few minutes and I was alarmed to hear that it was going to take some time.

'Now, as you will appreciate,' Dr MacKean continued, 'I am not able to disclose to you all my findings; they are confidential between me and the insurance company though naturally, if there is something wrong with you which needs treatment I will tell you about it. The insurance company have sent me a form to fill in so we will work our way steadily through it. I have your full name and address, nationality, date and place of birth, and will just enter this onto the form.'

He took out an old black fountain pen and, after shaking it furiously to get the ink to flow, he started writing slowly and deliberately. The old joke about doctors' handwriting being illegible came into my mind and I could see that there was considerable truth in it. His pen scratched a blotchy entry into the first box on the front of the form.

'Now we come to the questions, Justin. The first one asks about your dental health. How are your teeth?'

'I'm a dentist, so they should be all right.'

'Well, yes, they should, but just because a fellow is a motor mechanic doesn't necessarily mean his car never goes wrong. You had better let me take a look. I don't have a fancy inspection lamp like you chaps, so I use this.'

He swung round the battered old angle-poise lamp on his desk and directed it at my mouth. He then produced a mouth mirror from a drawer, which was so scratched and misty it would have been impossible to see much through it.

'Old Mr Padginton gave me this some years ago. Now open wide. Mm. It looks as if you've got a cavity down there.'

'Down where?' I demanded indignantly. I was a bit peeved that he was carrying out an examination of my teeth anyway. I felt that, in the circumstances he should have taken my word for it when I said they were all right. I also felt fairly strongly that doctors in general knew very little about dentistry and, having had my teeth checked by one of my colleagues just before I left university, I was quite certain there weren't any cavities.

'Bottom left six'.

'It can't be. I had the six extracted when I was nine years old. It must be the seven and I know what you are looking at. The area you think is a cavity is simply staining in a fissure.'

'It looks like a cavity to me,' persisted Dr MacKean. 'It's definitely brown.'

'I know its brown,' I retorted sharply, 'but that doesn't make it a cavity. If you examined it with a probe you would find that it is perfectly hard. A brown area on a tooth is not necessarily decay and it only needs to be treated if it's soft. I know that this particular area is fine. The staining has been present for many years, it has been checked many times, and it isn't a cavity.'

'Well I suppose you should know,' shrugged Dr MacKean who continued with his dental examination.

'It definitely looks as if there is a cavity at this side.'

'You mean upper right five?'

'Yes, there is a gap at the side of a filling.'

'I know there is, but it's all right.'

'What do you mean it's all right? You can't go around with holes in your teeth. You must get that filling replaced right away.'

'It's an experiment.' I explained. 'The tooth has been filled with a new type of white filling material that isn't yet in general use. One of my tutors placed the filling two years ago and we want to see how it wears over a three year period. As you can see it obviously isn't as strong as amalgam because some of it has chipped away, but we don't want to remove it yet because the three years isn't up.'

'And meanwhile you go around with a hole in your tooth?' Dr MacKean looked horrified. 'I always thought that if you didn't get holes filled up you were asking for trouble.'

'Depends on the hole. As long as there's no decay it won't come to any harm as long as it is kept clean.'

'Well, I never,' huffed Dr MacKean, 'opinions do change as time goes by. They are constantly changing in medicine. I can hardly keep up with it. I suppose I had better leave dentistry to you chaps and get on with the rest of your medical. Take off your shirt and let me listen to your heart.'

I did as he requested and stood upright whilst Dr MacKean and his stethoscope carried out an extremely thorough investigation.

'Breathe in and out. In and out. Mm... and again... mm. Hold it.'

All the time he was listening his tongue was pushing out his lower lip and his jowls appeared to become more pronounced. The concentration on his face was quite alarming and his examination seemed to go on for an eternity. In the end I began to think he had discovered a heart or lung defect and was trying to pin it down. Surely no ordinary examination could possibly take this long. Finally he put down his stethoscope and wrote something on the insurance form.

'Now I want you on the couch.'

He spread the blanket over the cold leather and invited me to jump up. The couch was quite high so I turned my back to it, placed both hands on it and gave myself a quick hoist upwards. As soon as my bottom touched down, the blanket glided over the slippery leather surface. Dr MacKean stood watching helplessly as I shot past him and made an unexpected and painful close inspection of the green linoleum.

'Are you all right, Justin?' cried Dr MacKean as he anxiously rushed to my assistance. 'I should have warned you about that; it is a positive death-trap.'

'It certainly is.' I rose to my feet rubbing my elbow, which seemed to be the part of me to have come off worst.

'Are you sure you're all right? Let me look at your elbow.'

'I'm all right, thank you.'

I went back to the couch and very carefully raised myself up on to it. I wondered how many other patients had come to grief in exactly the same way. He really ought to do something about that; it was downright dangerous. He was likely to get sued by someone. I could just imagine someone going to see the doctor for a minor complaint and coming away with a broken arm.

Once on the couch, Dr MacKean set about testing my reflexes. Out came his little rubber hammer and I was tapped in the most unlikely places whilst all he said was 'mm.'

He checked my blood pressure, which produced more thrusting forward of his lower lip, more 'mms' and more writing on the form. After a lot of prodding and poking as I lay on the couch he said, 'jump down now, Justin, and I'll check your height and weight.'

Dismounting from the couch was almost as hazardous as getting on it, but I was now wise to the problem and made sure that I accomplished it without mishap.

Dr MacKean's weighing machine was of similar vintage to his couch. It resembled conventional bathroom scales but his had an extra-large circular dial with a pointer. When I stood on the scales the pointer behaved like the speedometer on a Morris Minor. Anyone who has ever owned a Morris Minor will be familiar with the violent fluctuations of the needle. I thought at first that perhaps I wasn't standing perfectly still and I tried desperately hard not to move. However, try as I may I could not stop the pointer from moving about. After watching the dial for some time Dr MacKean announced that my weight was somewhere between eight and thirteen stone, but he couldn't be more precise than that.

'Do you know your weight?' he asked.

'I think it was about nine and a half stone last time I weighed myself, but that was some time ago.'

'Nine and a half stone sounds about right. You are quite skinny, aren't you? I'll put that on the form. How tall are you?'

'Five foot eight, I think.'

'I'll take your word for that too. The arm on my height gauge is a bit bent, so I have to add about an inch and a quarter to the reading to get an accurate measurement but it's a bit hit and miss like the scales.'

Dr MacKean wrote down the figures and turned the page. 'Still a fair way to go.'

His statement provided an answer to the question that was in my mind at that moment. I was wondering how much longer the examination would take. Spencer had said that he thought it would be brief and straightforward. He had certainly been wrong about that.

'I need to test your eyes now. Go and stand over there with your back against the door and face the chart.'

I did as Dr MacKean requested. I had always considered that I had very good eyesight, though I had never actually undergone an eye test. After all, it would have been difficult to carry out dentistry with defective vision and I was also able to see distant objects very clearly. I felt sure that I would pass this test with flying colours. However, when I looked at Dr MacKean's chart I realised that things might not be quite as straightforward as I had first thought.

The chart itself was so old that instead of there being clear black letters against a clean white background, age had darkened the whole of the chart to a dirty, yellowish brown, thus reducing the overall contrast. To make matters worse, there were what looked like tea or coffee stains all over it. And in addition, the illumination provided by the single, feeble light bulb was extremely limited.

Dr MacKean put his hand over my right eye. 'Can you read the next to bottom line on the chart, Justin?'

I read out the letters with some hesitation and, at times, a certain amount of guesswork.

Dr MacKean did not comment on my performance but moved his hand to cover up my left eye. 'Now can you read the bottom line?'

This presented me with considerably more difficulty and I used a lot more guesswork in making out the letters.

'Mm,' said Dr MacKean. 'Can you read the second letter on the next to bottom line, and the last two letters on that line?' All the time Dr MacKean was leaning forward lifting his own glasses up and down as he tried to make out the letters. Then he held his glasses some four inches in front of his face as if he were looking through a pair of binoculars.

'Mm, full marks with your left eye but your right eye's not quite as good. I suppose your eyes aren't too bad really, considering that the light in here isn't very bright.'

'No it isn't, and your chart isn't as clear as it might be.'

'That's true, but it is a few years old.'

'Yes, I can see that. But if you stand where I'm standing and cover up one eye how much can *you* read?' As I said it I realised it sounded a bit impertinent, but I didn't feel the test was very satisfactory. I was sure my eyesight was pretty good and I didn't want Dr MacKean writing anything on the form which would indicate otherwise. I don't know what he did write, but he spent a few minutes scratching away with his pen. I tried to look over his shoulder but his writing was difficult enough to read when it was right in front of you, so it was impossible to decipher from a distance.

Dr MacKean's next move was to take out his auroscope and he spent what seemed like an eternity looking into my ears, then he looked up my nose, down my throat, and in my hair.

'Not much further to go now, Justin. Will you please slip off your trousers so that I can check that you haven't got piles?'

'Piles? I haven't got piles. I can assure you I haven't.'

'I'm sure you haven't, but I have to check. Just to be absolutely certain.'

'I am absolutely certain.' I echoed adamantly.

'Come now, Justin, you know I can't fill in the form unless I have checked everything for myself. It won't take a minute. I'll examine you for a hernia at the same time.'

'Hernia!' I spluttered in disbelief, 'anything else?'

'Well I really ought to check you for prostate trouble, but I think you are probably a bit young for that so we can give that one a miss.'

'Thank heaven for that.'

'I must, however, satisfy myself that you haven't got varicose veins. I understand it is an occupational hazard for dentists.'

'Varicose veins? This is ridiculous. I've only been in general practice a few weeks – it's hardly long enough to have caused me to develop varicose veins.'

'I merely remarked that a lot of dentists do get varicose veins because their job involves standing on their feet for long periods. I wasn't suggesting that dentistry might have given them to you. I don't expect you have varicose veins, though it's not unknown for quite young people to get them, and, as I said to you before, I cannot fill in the form unless I have checked for myself.'

I suddenly felt that Dr MacKean was displaying enormous patience and I wasn't being at all cooperative. In the end I decided that I had better get it over with as quickly as possible so, in spite of overwhelming embarrassment, I removed my remaining items of clothing.

Dr MacKean was mercifully swift in completing this part of the examination and his years of experience as a doctor ensured that it was carried out with a professional detachment, which helped to some extent to allay my feelings of humiliation.

'Right, Justin, you can get dressed now. That takes care of everything.'

I was delighted to hear it. The whole thing had turned out to be a tremendous ordeal and I couldn't get my clothes back on fast enough.

'Well,' said Dr MacKean, 'as I told you earlier, I am not allowed to discuss my findings in detail but I don't think you will have any trouble getting your insurance.'

'So I am not in need of medical attention then, Dr MacKean?'

'No, I don't think so. In fact hopefully you won't be for another thirty or forty years.'

'I am pleased and relieved to hear it, and thank you for being patient with me. As you probably gathered, medical examinations are not my favourite pastime.'

'They are popular with very few people, Justin, but unfortunately they are a necessary evil from time to time.'

Dr MacKean showed me to the door. 'Take care, Justin, it has been nice meeting you. Perhaps we can meet again sometime under more pleasant circumstances; for you I mean. I hope you will enjoy working with Spencer Padginton.'

CHAPTER SEVENTEEN

Ever since Anna's leaving party I had felt guilty about letting down Richard Darcy, especially as he had been kind enough to invite me out with him. I appreciated the fact that he realised I didn't know many people because I was new to the area, and I was grateful that he was prepared to take the trouble to help me integrate into the Luccombury society.

He had been very understanding when I phoned to cancel our meeting, despite the fact that it had been at short notice. I didn't want him to think that I wasn't interested in seeing him and I had, in fact spoken to him twice on the phone since then.

We had finally made another arrangement to go out together and I had managed to find his house without any difficulty. I parked my car outside his white painted wrought iron garden gate. I was immediately drawn to the pocket handkerchief-sized lawn in his tiny but immaculate front garden. It was completely weed-free and every blade of grass was uniformly trimmed to a height of one inch. Just one or two relatively bare patches prevented it from being perfect. The overall effect of the garden, however, was quite impressive but not half as impressive as the sheer volume of the music that was rattling the windows inside his house. It was a heavy classical piece, which I didn't recognise, though this was hardly surprising since, although I enjoyed classical music and was becoming more interested in it, my knowledge of it was still fairly limited.

I wondered how he could possibly hear his doorbell, but he did, and soon appeared at the door looking slightly harassed.

'Hello,' he smiled, 'come in and sit down. I'm running a bit late I'm afraid, the phone hasn't stopped ringing since I got in from work.' He sensed that I was having difficulty hearing him above the music. 'Hang on I'll turn it down ... Mahler,' he revealed before I had time to ask.

He went over to the amplifier but instead of turning it down he turned it up. 'Just listen to this bit, it's fantastic.' He began conducting with wild and exaggerated flourishes of the arms.

'Cor,' he extolled, finally turning down the volume to an acceptable level. 'Did you hear how the horns built up to a crescendo? This, I think, is the liveliest recording of this piece I have ever heard. It's taken a little bit faster than usual, but I think that's greatly to its advantage. Don't you think so?'

'I'm afraid I don't know Mahler well enough to be able to give an opinion,' I replied truthfully.

'It's brilliant. I love Mahler. I always try out a new girlfriend with Mahler's Fourth. If she doesn't like it, I think there will be very little chance I shall be able to get on with her.'

'How many girls have you met who do like it?' I asked, thinking it highly unlikely that the average girl's taste in music would extend that far.

'Well, actually, only one and she was a professional violinist.'

'What happened to her? I assume that you're not still together.'

'No, it didn't work out long term. Lasted about two months as I recall.'

'So a liking for Mahler is not enough on its own?'

'No, but it's a start and fairly essential. But the search goes on. Who knows? – tonight I might be lucky and find the girl of my dreams.'

Everything in the house from the furniture to the decorations looked about twenty years out of date. It was detached though there was only about a three-foot gap between each of the houses on the street. It was of modest proportions and with the classic design of stairs facing the front door with bathroom above the entrance hall, kitchen at the rear and two reception rooms which, in Richard's house, had been made into one long room. The carpet and three piece suite were brightly coloured and of a floral pattern. It was very clean and tidy but there was an overwhelming feeling of it being terribly old-fashioned. I have to say that it was not a bit like I expected the bachelor home of a dynamic young solicitor to be.

'Where had you planned on going this evening?' I asked.

'I have a carefully planned itinerary. I always go down to the coast, as there isn't much going on around here. There are two or three places I try first. I vary the order depending on what day it is. One of the places is particularly good on Wednesday evenings because the girls from a local insurance office all meet up there before going on to a night club. Friday night is good at another place just after ten, because a group of girls go in there after their evening classes finish at the local college. The French class were in there last week so I was able to give them a little bit of extra tuition. Teach them some of the things they're not likely to learn in a classroom, but without which they would be unable to face the big wide world fully educated and prepared.'

His eyes glinted as he spoke.

'I take it you can speak French then?'

'Oh yes, fluently. I studied French Law at Oxford as part of my degree and spent six months over there. My German is pretty good too, but not quite as good as my French. Now, I thought tonight we might kick off by trying a new wine bar that has just opened up. I've heard quite good reports about the type of talent that has been seen frequenting it. Things are completely different at this time of year from the height of the holiday season. Everywhere gets very crowded in the summer and there's nothing worse than meeting some cracking looking bit of stuff only to find that she's here on holiday and that she'll be going back to Runcorn at the weekend.'

'How often do you go out looking for girls?'

'Every night, unless of course I'm taking one out. Though that doesn't necessarily stop me looking.'

'Do you have any other interests?' I asked somewhat intrigued by Richard's apparent single mindedness.

'Other than looking for women? No, not really, except for my love of classical music. What about you? Have you been up to anything interesting recently?'

'No. I'm still trying to get myself organised in the cottage I'm renting. The most exciting thing I have done this week was to go for an insurance medical. It was quite an experience, I can tell you.'

'Who did you see? Don't tell me... Dr MacKean.'

'That's right, how did you know?'

'Well, there are only two doctors around here so I had a fifty percent chance of being right anyway, and in any case, I happen to know that he tends to specialise in insurance medicals. Makes quite a bit of beer money from it I understand. That and ash cash.'

'Ash cash?'

'Yes, haven't you heard of it? If someone who's croaked is going to be cremated, there has to be a second doctor to sign the death certificate. He gets a nice little fee for the service. I don't know how much, but it's pretty easy money by the sound of it. All he has to do is go and take a look at the stiff and sign the certificate.'

'Do you know Dr MacKean?'

'Yeah, he's my doctor. I go to his surgery once a year for a check-up. I was there only a couple of weeks ago. He's just got a new nurse. Not bad, actually. I think if it went to the Court of Appeal the appeal would be upheld.'

I didn't fully understand the reference to the legal process, but it was obviously his way of saying that she was attractive. He continued. 'MacKean got her to take my blood pressure, weigh me and fill in a questionnaire. She asked me if I played any sport or did any swimming. I said I didn't. She then asked what I did for exercise. I said, "I flirt". She wasn't a bit amused and with a completely deadpan expression she said, "there isn't much exercise in that." To which I replied, " there is if my flirting is successful". She still wasn't amused. Shame she had no sense of humour. She struck me as the sort of girl you could take to your parents' house for Sunday lunch, unlike most of the girls I seem to meet these days. Know what I mean?

'She told me I had high blood pressure. I said, "well what do you expect standing so close to me and squeezing the bulb on your sphygmomanometer, or whatever you call it, in such a provocative way? It's enough to give any young man high blood pressure". Anyway, I got MacKean to check it again a few days later because it did worry me a bit that my blood pressure might be high. Fortunately it was back to normal then so she must have had some effect on me.'

Suddenly Richard jumped up, leapt over to the hi-fi system and turned up the volume to a deafening level. 'Listen to this bit, it's superb.' He began conducting the orchestra once more. 'Cor, that's fantastic,' he enthused after he had returned the volume to a more normal level.

'It's a nice house, Richard. How long have you had it?'

'About two and a half years. It belonged to my grandfather, so I got it relatively cheaply. It was in a bit of a state and I've spent some money on it.'

'Did you do your own decorating?'

'No, but I was going to. I started in the main bedroom; I took a week off work to do it. At the end of the week I still hadn't stripped the wallpaper off one wall. I realised it was going to take forever, and it was then I decided to call in the professionals. They fitted out the kitchen and bathroom and decorated throughout. I got them to knock down the wall between the sitting room and the dining room to make one big room, and they fitted the patio door. They had props everywhere holding up the walls and floor upstairs. I was wetting myself that the whole house was going to collapse. I thought when they knocked down a wall they did it gently brick by brick. I couldn't believe it when this eighteen stone tattooed thicko picked up a damn great sledge hammer and started knocking hell out of it.'

'What did you say?'

'Say? I didn't say anything. I got out quick in case the whole house came down. Discretion is the b...b...b...better part of v...v...valour,' he stammered, impersonating Ronnie Barker's portrayal of Arkwright, the shopkeeper, in the TV series *Open All Hours*. 'That was enough for me. I moved out and went to stay with my mother until all the work was finished. It took them just over four weeks but they did a good job, don't you think?'

'Yes, they did.' I agreed. I felt that the wallpaper and carpets would not have been my choice, but I didn't say so.

The house was probably built in the 1940s and whilst it was solid and comfortable it was definitely lacking in character and Richard's choice of decoration did little to improve it. There was a beige coloured regency striped wallpaper in the sitting room and a deeply embossed fleur-de- lis pattern paper of a similar colour in the hall. The balusters on the staircase had been boxed in with hardboard, which was painted brilliant white like all the other woodwork in the house. The tiny kitchen was pale lilac and had light oak effect wall cupboards. All the ceilings were papered with Anaglypta paper and painted white and in the centre of every ceiling there hung a pendant light fitting. The carpets were a different colour in every room with little thought given to continuity. They were all verging on being gaudy, and the brightly coloured suite in the sitting room clashed terribly with the carpet.

Richard looked at his watch. 'I'd better get a move on, it's time we went. We really need to be at the Lord Nelson before nine o'clock. That's the time the yobs start arriving. If there is any unattached crumpet of any merit we need to be there to snap it up before they arrive. I was just drying my hair when you came. I think it's important not to go out with wet hair, don't you think? I don't want to catch cold.'

'You won't catch cold. I often wash my hair and go out straight away without drying it. It's quite mild out anyway.'

He disappeared upstairs and left me with the evening paper. I could hear his hairdryer for several minutes, followed by a long spell of silence. The record had finished playing, there was very little through traffic along the road outside and suddenly it was remarkably peaceful. I sat there thinking that I would be quite content to stay in and read occasionally if I lived there, unlike Richard for whom the quest for women appeared to take priority over everything else.

Finally he appeared and announced that he was ready to go out.

'I must just turn everything off and make sure it's safe. You can't be too c...c...c...careful,' he said, repeating his Ronnie Barker stammer.

'Move out into the hall, Justin, I need a clear area to make sure that everything is turned off. I start at the doorway and work clockwise round the room from there.'

He went to each power point in turn pulling out the plugs. 'Now, that's off, that's off,' he said out loud each time he pulled out a plug. 'That's off.'

When he had gone all the way round the room he then went round a second time checking that he hadn't missed any plugs. As he inspected each power point he once more declared out loud, 'that's definitely off, definitely off.'

Having satisfied himself that all was safe, he locked the door to the sitting room and removed the key. 'Now I'll check the kitchen,' he said and started to go through the same ritual with all the power points in there. When he had done this he turned his attention to the gas cooker. 'That's off, off, off, off, off,' he recited as he worked his way three times along the row of knobs on the control panel. Next he went to the fridge and pushed the door so hard the whole fridge rocked. He did this five or six times and finally declared, 'that's off.'

'A fridge can catch fire you know if the door isn't closed. The compressor works overtime trying to keep the temperature down and as a result it overheats,' he explained to me pushing the door once more to be absolutely certain. 'It's definitely off, isn't it?'

'The door is closed, if that's what you mean,' I replied somewhat superciliously. 'But it was closed in the first place.'

'I know but you can't be too c...c...careful.'

I had watched him in utter amazement as he had gone through the routine of checking that everything was safe. Being careful was one thing, but I saw this as being obsessional.

'I'll just get my coat and we'll go.'

He was already wearing a jacket which, given the temperature, I considered to be adequate, bearing in mind that we probably weren't going be outside for any length of time. Richard, however, came back putting on a well-worn anorak and a woollen scarf.

'Right,' he said, ' we'll be off.'

He followed me outside and locked the front door. After taking the key from the lock he put his shoulder against the door and pushed hard to check that it was secure. One push wasn't enough, of course, to satisfy him that it was properly locked and he stood there for nearly two minutes and must have pushed it at least twenty times.

'By the time you've gone through all the business of checking that everything is safe it'll be too late to go anywhere,' I said somewhat sarcastically.

He wasn't at all offended by my remark. 'I didn't get where I am today without checking everything thoroughly before going out.' I realised that this expression also came from some television series. As he had told me that he went out virtually every evening, I wondered how he managed to watch television but he obviously did, and appeared to be a keen fan of quite a few comedy programmes.

'As I said before,' he continued, 'you can't be...'

'I know, too c...c...c...careful,' I interrupted.

'Precisely,' he nodded with a smile.

I was rapidly reaching the conclusion that he was totally eccentric, but nevertheless there was something quite likeable about him.

'We'd better go in my car,' he exclaimed when he saw that I had a sports car. 'If we pick something up there won't be room in yours.'

CHAPTER EIGHTEEN

It was surprisingly warm inside his car and instinctively I opened the window a small amount.

'Don't open the window,' Richard exclaimed with alarm. 'I don't want to be in a draught.'

I immediately wound it back up again.

We covered the twelve or so miles to the coast at a very modest pace.

'Just look at that red Rover; that's a diabolical piece of driving,' Richard cried. 'He deserves to have the book thrown at him. Did you see how he overtook that Mini? He couldn't possibly see over the brow of the hill, he couldn't have known whether it was clear or not. He was doing about eighty when he overtook me. If I could catch up with him, I'd perform a citizen's arrest.'

There was no danger of Richard ever being stopped for speeding; every road sign and speed limit was obeyed instantly and absolutely. In that sense he was a very good driver.

'I have to be very careful in my position, you know, Justin. I have to keep my nose clean. It would be unthinkable for me to be convicted of any sort of criminal offence, even a minor motoring offence. I must make sure that no-one is allowed to have any sort of hold over me.'

At that moment a yellow Ford Capri came zooming up behind us and, as there was no possibility of it being able to overtake at that moment, he stayed behind us only a matter of a few feet from Richard's rear bumper.

'Just look at that idiot behind us,' gasped Richard, 'look how close he is.'

We had been travelling at about forty miles per hour but Richard slowed right down. The Ford Capri had no alternative but to slow down also, though at one point he very nearly touched our bumper. Richard slowed to about ten miles per hour to the intense annoyance of the Ford driver who was leaning hard on his horn.

'Just listen to the blasted idiot,' scoffed Richard, 'typical bloody Ford Capri driver. It is my policy when people follow too closely to slow right down to a speed that will allow them to stop within the distance between our cars. The closer they get the slower I go.'

It was a policy that wasn't exactly endearing him to the Ford driver who was still blowing his horn as well as flashing his headlights and shaking his fist. I thought at one point that he was about to ram us from behind. Fortunately, the road straightened out and widened and the Ford pulled out and set off past us like a greyhound out of the trap. Suddenly he cut in across the front of Richard's car, missing the offside front corner by a whisker, and causing Richard to brake sharply and swerve away.

'The bloody idiot. People like that shouldn't be on the road,' cursed Richard as he watched the Ford rapidly disappear into the distance ahead of him.

The rest of the journey was less eventful and we arrived at the car park of the Lord Nelson. It was quite busy and we drove round several times before we found a space where Richard was happy to leave his car. It was right at the back of the car park and some considerable distance from the building.

'I'm very fussy who I park next to. I would never park next to a Ford Capri for example. The thicko we encountered on the way here just proves my case. I don't want to come back and find my door smashed in.'

Richard took off his scarf and anorak and locked them in the boot. He then went round checking that all the doors were locked. My assurance that my door was locked was not good enough for him and he insisted on checking it for himself and, in fact, walked round the car three times pulling at each door handle before he was satisfied.

As we walked across the car park, Richard buttoned up his jacket and turned up his collar. 'It's quite chilly, isn't it? You don't think I'll catch cold do you?'

'I shouldn't think so; the fresh air will do you good. You probably don't get enough in your job being stuck in an office all day.' Richard said nothing and looked unconvinced.

The Lord Nelson was quite a large building and as we approached the entrance, live music greeted us. 'That's the Bigwoods you can hear,' Richard explained. 'They play here three nights a week in the bar on the right just inside the entrance. Downstairs is Donna Black on piano; she's been playing here regularly for years. We'll go and see her in a minute if we don't strike lucky upstairs. There are five separate bars and I usually visit each one in strict rotation to see what's about, though I have had considerably more lucky strikes in the first bar than in any of the others.'

I assumed that by 'lucky strikes' he referred to picking up girls. I personally had never 'picked up' a girl in my life but I did not admit this to Richard. To be honest I didn't really know how to go about it. I thought it was most unlikely that I would be brave enough to wander over to a complete stranger in a pub and start chatting her up. I was much too shy for that. In the event, I said nothing and followed Richard inside.

The first bar we visited where the Bigwoods were playing was a large room, very crowded and extremely smoky. The music was deafening and we had to shout at each other. Richard knew quite a few other young men who were obviously there for the same reason as him. He said 'Hello' and exchanged the odd word or two but neither he nor they seemed interested in getting involved in conversation though one tall, dark-haired young man wearing jeans and a T-shirt seemed to want to be friendly and offered to buy Richard a drink. Richard's abrupt refusal was less than polite and he promptly walked away. 'You have to be so careful in my position,' he said seriously. 'If someone saw me accepting a drink it might be construed as a bribe.'

'Surely there's no harm in letting someone buy you a drink,' I returned, thinking that Richard's cautiousness was now verging on the ridiculous. 'Does that mean I can't buy you a drink?'

'That's different. You are a professional man and a friend. It's casual acquaintances wearing an earring and training shoes that I worry about. As I've said before 'you c...c...c...can't be too c...c...c...careful. In any case, I don't like being with more than one person when I go out. If there are just two of you, it's easy to split up two girls who are out together, but if there are more than two of you, they see you as being out in a gang and somehow it becomes more difficult. They don't seem so receptive. My friend John phoned me up to see if I would go out with him this evening but as I had arranged to meet you I told him I couldn't.'

I took this as another lesson from Richard in the art of picking up women. I obviously had a great deal to learn.

Richard's eyes scanned the room from one end to the other and he was constantly craning his neck peering through the gaps in the crowd in the hope of spotting an unattached female. His entire surveillance operation took about five minutes. 'There's nothing any good here, let's adjourn to the next bar.'

'Do you want a drink?' I asked.

'We'll get one later, let's move on.'

The next bar we went into was smaller and much quieter, the lighting was more subdued and although it was quite busy, most people were sitting at tables unlike the last bar where everyone was standing.

'Do you want to sit down and I'll get us a drink,'

'Good Lord, no,' exclaimed Richard. 'I never sit down. I like to keep on the move so that I don't miss anything. We could go and get a drink and stand at the bar if you like.'

'What do you drink?'

'G and T, please,' said Richard.

'Do you want a double?'

'No, no. I never have more than one single gin in an evening.'

I ordered his gin and tonic and a pint of beer for myself. I was about to take my first drink when suddenly Richard exclaimed, 'quick, let's adjourn to the bar opposite. I've just seen some promising crumpet go in there.'

I was unceremoniously pushed towards the door spilling my drink as I went. Richard didn't even bother to take his drink with him.

'Cor, look at that,' exploded Richard as we entered another small bar very similar in style to the last one. 'Look at the tall blonde over there. I haven't seen her in here before. God, she's certainly well put together. I would most definitely allow the appeal on that one; I would have no hesitation in taking that to the

Court of Appeal. In fact, I would go so far as to say I would be prepared to take it to the House of Lords.'

'So what do we do now, then?' I asked innocently, wondering what Richard's next move would be.

'We just wait here and watch. I am sure she looked this way a minute ago. She'll probably look again soon if she's interested. There did you see that? I'm sure I got a sign then.'

'I didn't see anything.' I replied truthfully.

'I'm quite certain of it,' insisted Richard. 'Watch carefully, I'm sure she's interested.

The girl in question was standing with two others and a curly haired man. She was talking to all three of them but mainly to the man who had his back to us. This meant she was facing our way but so far I hadn't seen her look beyond the man. It seemed to me that it was him she was interested in.

'Perhaps that's her boyfriend,' I suggested.

'No, she's not the slightest bit interested in him,' said Richard, 'you can see that quite clearly.'

'The girl in blue, with her, looks quite nice,' I offered thinking that if and when Richard made his move I might be forced to go with him and try my hand at chatting up one of them.

'She looks okay but I suspect it's U.S.I.,' returned Richard.

'U.S.I?'

'Unlawful sexual intercourse – under sixteen. The tall blonde isn't U.S.I., though. I reckon she could teach even me a thing or two.'

'What makes you say that?' I asked, absolutely intrigued that Richard could apparently tell so much about a girl he had seen for only a few minutes at a distance of some ten yards and had never even spoken to.

'You can tell these things when you have had some experience. Look, I definitely got a flicker then. Did you see it? No doubt about it that time. One more and I shall have to move in on her.'

I still failed to see that she was looking at anyone other than the man she was talking to but Richard seemed sure of himself. I was longing to know how he would go about making himself known to her.

'Are you going to offer to buy her a drink?'

'Certainly not. I didn't get where I am today by shelling out good money on women in pubs. There she looked then, did you see it that time?'

'Well, to be perfectly honest, I can't say that I did. I saw her smile but it looked to me as though she smiled at the man she's talking to.'

'With the greatest respect, M'Lud, the man she is talking to is a wally. I've told you, she isn't the slightest bit interested in him. Just look at him; training shoes and an earring, just like all of the other wallies in here. I wouldn't grant bail to anyone wearing training shoes and definitely not if he's wearing an earring as well. Would you grant him bail?'

'He looks all right to me. A bit scruffy maybe, but he's okay.'

'Members of the jury, my learned friend has admitted that the defendant looked "a bit scruffy". No doubt you will draw your own conclusions from that. Justin, what would a clean, smart, cracking looking bit of stuff like her want with an earring wearing thicko like him when there are fellows like me around? There I rest my case.'

At that moment the group of four suddenly made their way to the door.

'Quick, come on,' snapped Richard, 'we can't let that escape.'

We set off after them at something considerably less than a discrete distance, and finished up back in the first bar where the Bigwoods were still making conversation impossible except by shouting. Richard took up a strategic position some ten yards away from where the blonde girl and her friends were standing.

'There, I told you it wasn't her boyfriend,' shouted Richard in my ear. 'She's ignoring him now and talking to the girl in blue. If they play a slow number I'm going to ask her for a dance.'

As it happened the next number was slow. Richard jumped into action. 'Right, here we go'

He strode boldly over to her and I moved in a little closer in the hope of being able to hear what was said. Luckily the reduction in tempo was accompanied by a corresponding reduction in volume.

'Excuse me, my dear, I was wondering whether you would be so good as to do me the honour of treading a measure with me?'

'What?' came the reply and the girl screwed up her face in puzzlement.

'I was wondering whether you would care to dance with me,' explained Richard.

'No thank you.'

'Well, that is a bitter disappointment but perhaps then, you would do me the honour of allowing me to engage in polite conversation with you for a few minutes. You look like a very bright, intelligent and interesting person, not to mention your great beauty. It is rare, indeed to meet people like you these days. I find that people generally are so dull and ill-mannered with little common sense and totally lacking in social graces. I knew as soon as I saw you that you possess that certain *je ne sais quoi* and that you were a person I really wanted to meet.'

'You're certainly a smooth talker, I'll give you that,' replied the girl laughing.

'I have to be in my job, but that's not to say that I didn't mean what I said.'

'So what is your job?'

'I'm a solicitor. Richard Lindsay Darcy at your service, madam.'

He held out his hand and the girl offered her hand in return. Richard kissed it, bowing as he did so.

'I am your man if you need legal representation, an expert in divorce law. I do some conveyancing but it isn't really my scene I prefer to be in court grappling with something juicy.'

'I'm not having a divorce at the moment, thank you very much. I've been through all that, but it's all in the past now, thank goodness.'

'It can be very messy,' agreed Richard. 'I have acted in some very nasty cases. It is absolutely essential to have a good solicitor.'

'Where do you work?'

'In Luccombury.'

'Luccombury,' scoffed the girl. 'I wouldn't have thought you would get much work there as a high-powered solicitor; it's too quiet.'

'The town is quiet,' agreed Richard, 'but you would be amazed how busy I am most of the time, and I get my fair share of well-known celebrities seeking my services. Why only last week I received a call from … No, I shouldn't have started that – I am not at liberty to disclose any details. One of the first things I learnt after leaving Oxford University was that confidentiality must be maintained at all times. One cannot really discuss professional matters even with one's closest friends and relatives.'

'You were at Oxford university, were you?' said the girl.

'Yes, indeed I was. Balliol College. First class honours in English and French Law.

'Very impressive,' she said but sounding as though she was most unimpressed.

'I was wondering,' continued Richard, sensing that the slow number was coming to an end and that soon, conversation might become difficult again. 'Would you consider letting me take you out for a drink one evening, somewhere a little quieter than this?'

'I might,' she replied.

'If you let me have your name and telephone number I'll give you a bell in the next few days.' Richard produced a pen and paper and handed them to the girl who wrote something down and then handed them back to him. Richard returned them to his pocket, said something to the girl, which I couldn't hear and then came back to me, his face beaming.

'Her name's Shirley. I told you it wasn't her boyfriend, didn't I? I could tell she wasn't interested in him. She's cracking looking though, don't you think?'

'She is very attractive. Where does she live?'

'No idea.'

'Does she work?'

'Not a clue. All I know about her is that her name's Shirley, she's divorced, and she's cracking looking. I would definitely take the appeal to the House of Lords. She gave me her telephone number so I'll ring her tomorrow and arrange to take her out.'

'Do you think she'll come?'

'Yes, I think so, or she wouldn't have given me her telephone number.'

'Will you take her out to dinner?'

'Good Lord, no. I don't believe in shelling out too much on them on a first date. It will be a quick drink at a quiet country pub and then back to my place for the Mahler test. Come on, Justin, we might as well move on from here now; we aren't likely to strike lucky twice in the same place on the same night. I suggest we adjourn and try our luck at Frazer's Wine Bar. I've often seen some very spectacular-looking crumpet in there at about this time in the evening.'

I looked at him incredulously. 'Surely you aren't still looking, are you? Aren't you satisfied with the fact that you have effectively picked up one girl tonight?'

'Definitely not. You can't afford to stop looking; you never know what might be just round the corner. I believe in keeping my options open at all times and never stop looking. It has been a successful evening, in fact, the most successful evening for about two months. I was beginning to think the Lord Nelson wasn't worth visiting any more but it certainly was tonight. You obviously brought me luck – we shall have to go out together again. In the meantime let's go and see what we can find at Frazer's Wine Bar.'

CHAPTER NINETEEN

I decided that I had to talk to Spencer quite firmly about my nurse, or rather the fact that I still didn't have one. Daphne was supposed to be helping me in the surgery but the great problem was that she didn't get up until after eleven o'clock and, by the time she was ready for action, it was practically lunchtime. This meant that every day I had to look after myself for the entire morning. Having suffered this now for over a week, I made a point of arriving at the surgery a little bit earlier than usual, hoping that I might catch Spencer in the kitchen reading the newspaper, as he often did after breakfast. On this particular day, however, he wasn't there.

'Damn,' I thought, 'just when I really need to talk to him.'

I went up the stairs to my surgery to find that he was already up there, sitting at the desk in his surgery. He was poring over a huge chart which was spread out on top of all the patients' records and papers that permanently littered his desk. I went in to see him just as he was writing something on the chart; it appeared to be a graph of some sort.

'Oh, hello Justin. How are you today?'

'Fine thanks, Spencer. What are you doing?'

Spencer looked a bit sheepish. 'It's my weight chart,' he explained. 'I've been clapping on the pounds a bit recently and I have to lose some of it before my next holiday. As I tend to gain a bit when I'm away on holiday – well sometimes more than a bit – I have to prepare for it beforehand. It wouldn't be much of a holiday if I had to watch what I eat and drink. It looks from this chart that I need to lose about two stone over the next ten weeks.'

'That sounds a lot to me,' I said, thinking that it must be an awful nuisance to have to consider what you eat all the time. I had always been very slim – in fact, there were times when I wished I was a bit fatter – but I never seemed to put on any weight, and at least I could eat anything I wanted and not worry about it.

I looked at the graph and it was obvious that there had been a steady upward progression over the last few months. 'Do you keep a record of your weight all the time?'

'Yes, I weigh myself every morning after breakfast and enter it on the chart. It's the only way I can keep a proper check on it.'

Spencer took out a ruler, laid it on the chart and, using a red pen joined up the cross he was entering when I walked into his surgery, to yesterday's cross. There was no doubt the line was heading upwards.

'Doesn't look good, Spencer. It's gone up quite a bit in the last twenty-four hours. If you carry on at this rate you'll weigh twenty stone by the end of the month.'

'Daphne and I went to a dinner party last night so you can't really take too much notice of today's weight. I shall have very little to eat today, so tomorrow it will hopefully be back down again. It will be a concerted effort now, Justin. Over the next few weeks you will see the pounds just fall off me.'

Spencer folded his chart and placed it underneath the large blotting pad on his desk. He looked at my slim figure.

'You don't realise how lucky you are not having to think whether or not you can have an extra bit of cake or a second helping of pud. How much do you weigh?'

'Well according to Dr MacKean's scale I am somewhere between eight and thirteen stone, but he can't be more precise than that.'

'That sounds like old MacKean. How did you get on with him?'

'He put me through hell. You said it would be easy and that he wouldn't bother too much. You were wrong. I was there for ages; he checked absolutely everything and I mean everything.'

Spencer chuckled. 'I've heard about his insurance medicals before and that he is very thorough, which is a bit surprising because normally he is fairly laid back about things. He once said to me that when someone goes to see him he never bothers to examine them on the first visit; he simply takes their word for whatever they think is wrong with them. If they tell him they've got 'flu and need antibiotics, he simply writes a prescription for antibiotics and sends them on their way. If they say they've got a bad back and need painkillers, he gives them painkillers and doesn't even look at their back. For ninety percent of patients this works and they get better. If they go back a second time he then takes it a bit more seriously and has a look. Seems a bit risky to me, but that is the way he says he works.'

'There is a risk that someone might go to see him with something serious that needs instant attention.'

'I know. I am not sure I entirely believed him. I think, in actual fact, he is a wise old bird with years of experience. He has probably developed a sixth sense as to when he needs to take a patient seriously. I don't think much gets past him in spite of what he said. He didn't find anything wrong with you, then?'

'No I don't think so. I wouldn't have gone if I had known what he was going to put me through.'

'So he knows as much about you as any of the women in your life, eh Justin?'

'Considerably more, I would say. It was a most humiliating experience.'

'Medicals usually are. Well at least you will get your insurance cover and it will also have given you peace of mind that there is nothing wrong with you.'

'Peace of mind? I didn't think there was anything wrong with me anyway and, to be honest, I don't have much faith in doctors. I know someone who went for a medical exam, was passed fit and died of a heart attack on the way home. As for the insurance, I've decided not to go ahead with it.'

'What, after going through the medical?'

'That's what made my mind up for me. If I'm fit I won't need sickness insurance and I have come to the conclusion that insurance companies only like to take on safe bets so that they won't have to pay out. They went to a lot of trouble paying Dr MacKean to carry out a medical to make sure I was a safe bet before they accepted me. I was annoyed that their representative didn't tell me in the first place that I would have to have a medical. The premium will be quite expensive and I can't really afford it at present. No, my mind is made up. They can keep their sickness insurance.'

'I have never had any sickness insurance,' said Spencer. 'I never really felt it was worth it; I preferred to spend my money on beer and wine and other similar health giving products. I suppose if you did become ill you would be glad you had insurance to pay the bills whilst you aren't working, but I am happy to take my chances.'

'I really wanted to speak to you, Spencer, about your finding me a nurse. I can't go on much longer as I am at present.'

'I know, I know,' he agreed. 'I am sorry that you have had such a difficult time of it recently. Daphne's intentions were good when she offered to nurse for you, but we both know that she is not an early riser.'

'She's a good nurse when she's there, but she's never there in the mornings. It's very difficult to avoid running late when I have to do everything myself, and there are some jobs in dentistry that need two pairs of hands.'

'I wish I could get her out of bed at a reasonable time,' sighed Spencer, 'but I've been trying for years and I still haven't managed it. I thought that if I got her a dog it might encourage her to get up and take it for a walk, but I'm the one who has to take Dotty out.'

'I am absolutely shattered by the end of the morning. It gets so hectic trying to mix the filling material and then place it in the tooth on my own, and the worst part is clearing everything away ready for the next patient. It's no good for me and it's no good for the patients. What's worse is that I'm losing money because I'm not working efficiently.'

'I know,' Spencer agreed, 'we can't have that. If you are losing money then I'm losing money also. I have been trying hard to find you a nurse but there haven't been any suitable applicants – I didn't want a repeat of the episode with Sandra. As a matter of fact, there is a chance that I might have found someone for you. It's a German girl who came to England originally as an au pair, and she liked it so much she stayed here. She lives with a family who are patients of mine. They say she is very bright, clean, reliable and efficient.'

'Has she any previous dental nursing experience?'

'I don't think so, but if she's bright she'll soon pick it up. I'll phone up later and see if I can get her to come round here.'

'In the meantime, is there any chance of Daphne being up to help me this morning?'

'I shouldn't think so. As I said, we went to a dinner party last night. We didn't get back until after three; it was probably four o'clock before Daphne had taken off her make-up and finally got to bed.'

I groaned. 'I suppose I had better go and get myself organised for the first patient then,'

It was Mrs Gunn's big day today. The day her new gold denture was due to be fitted. She was booked in for half-past eleven and the denture had not yet been delivered from the laboratory where it was being made. I was a bit concerned that it still had not arrived; usually the work was delivered the day before it was actually needed.

The first part of the morning hadn't been too bad in spite of the fact that I had no nurse to help me. Most of the patients had been for routine check-ups and I could cope quite well with them on my own. At ten thirty, I decided that I ought to phone Melvyn, the dental technician, who was making Mrs Gunn's denture to check that it would arrive in time. There was no reply which indicated to me that he was probably on his way though I had no guarantee of that and no way of checking it.

Melvyn ran the local dental laboratory single-handed and worked extremely hard. A typical day for him began at six o'clock in the morning and he worked in his laboratory for about three hours before setting off on his first collection and delivery round. He would visit several dental surgeries in the area delivering dentures he had made or repaired for them and at the same time collect any new work. This took him until about eleven o'clock then he would work in his laboratory until three thirty or four o'clock before setting off on his second round of the dental surgeries. By visiting the surgeries twice in a day it meant that he was able to offer a same-day service for repairing dentures. As long as a patient handed in their denture to the surgery in time for Melvyn's first collection, it meant that they could have it back the same afternoon. It was a good service and much appreciated by patients but it placed great demands upon Melvyn. Very often he would go back to his laboratory in the evening and work late into the night. As his was a service that dentists relied upon heavily, he could have no time off work and hadn't had a single day's holiday since he established his business four years ago.

I had every confidence that he would not let me down but he was leaving it very late to deliver Mrs Gunn's denture. He finally arrived just before eleven fifteen, full of apologies. He had decided to give the denture a final polish before setting off on his round so he was later than usual and apparently the traffic had been heavy.

'I think you will be pleased with it, Justin,' he said proudly. He too admitted that he had never made a gold denture before so it was special to him also. He had put in a lot of extra effort to make it look really good.

'As long as it fits.' I said anxiously. Unfortunately there was no way of knowing whether it would or not. Every possible care had been taken with it but in spite of this, inaccuracies could creep in. The fit had to be perfect and if it wasn't there would be no alternative but to start all over again. Neither Melvyn nor I wanted that.

'Phone me up as soon as you know,' begged Melvyn, 'I can't bear to wait until I see you again this afternoon.'

'I'll phone and let you know as soon as I can.'

The denture did look magnificent, at least to a dentist's eyes. I had taken a lot of trouble with the impressions and spent an enormous amount of time choosing the shape, size and colour of the teeth that were fitted to it and making sure that they were in exactly the right position. It was clear that Melvyn had also put in a lot of effort.

I could hardly believe what I saw when I looked at Melvyn's bill for the denture. Most of the cost was, of course, in the gold itself. I decided that I ought to work out the total cost to Mrs Gunn so that I could have her account ready, just in case she wanted to settle it immediately. By the time I had included all the other treatment I had carried out for her the final bill amounted to £247 and a few pence. Spencer would, no doubt have simply charged 247 guineas, claiming it sounded more professional. I thought, however, that it would be too complicated to work out exactly how much 247 guineas was in pounds and pence, so I set the bill at £250 exactly, thinking this was a nice round sum. I didn't have time to type it so I wrote it out as neatly as I could and put it on my desk to await her arrival.

Mrs Gunn was early, as usual, but as the patient before her failed to attend I didn't have to keep her waiting. I was pleased about this because I was excited and also very apprehensive to the point that I had butterflies in my stomach.

'Good morning, Mrs Gunn, and how are you today?'

'I'm fine, Mr Derwent, thank you. Is today the day I can finally get rid of this old denture? Is my new one ready?'

'Yes, it is, Mrs Gunn, and it looks wonderful. I am sure you will be very pleased with it.'

'I'm so happy, Mr Derwent. Come on then don't keep me in suspense any longer.' She clapped her hands together and bounced up and down like an impatient schoolgirl.

Very slowly I placed the denture in her mouth and applied gentle pressure to seat it into position. It slid home like a dream.

Thank you, Melvyn, thank you. You have done a first class job, I thought to myself. All the care and trouble had paid off.

'It fits beautifully, Mrs Gunn.'

'It feels marvellous, Mr Derwent. It's a bit different from my old one, but I know I shall get used to it very quickly. I can just tell I will. How does it look?'

I handed her a mirror and she examined herself closely. 'It looks extremely natural and matches my own teeth perfectly. No-one would ever know that I am wearing a denture. You are brilliant, Mr Derwent, quite brilliant.'

I felt just as delighted and more than a little relieved. 'I am so pleased you like it Mrs Gunn. It is possible, of course, that you might need a slight adjustment; we shan't know until you have tried eating with it. I suggest that you go home and see how you get on with it and let me know if you need any help.'

'I'll test it on a nice juicy steak, Mr Derwent.'

'Good idea, but make sure it isn't too tough.'

'Oh I get my meat from the local butcher, Mr Savage. He always gives me tender steaks. His meat is always very good. Now, Mr Derwent you must let me have your account. You have worked very hard and you deserve to be paid. Do you want to send it to me or shall I settle up with you now?'

'It's entirely up to you, Mrs Gunn, I will send it to you if you like, though I do have it here ready if you would prefer to deal with it now.'

'In that case, I will settle it right away. It will save the postage and it will all be over and done with so I can forget about it. I don't like owing people money.'

I handed her my hand-written account. She looked at it carefully for a few moments.

'You silly boy,' she laughed, 'you have added a nought by mistake. You quite frightened me for a moment, Mr Derwent.'

'Have I, Mrs Gunn? How careless of me. I am sorry but I prepared it in rather a hurry. Give it back to me and I'll alter it for you.'

I took the bill from her and looked at the figures, then I looked at her again. Suddenly I smiled at her. 'You're pulling my leg, Mrs Gunn. You are trying to wind me up, aren't you?'

Slowly my smile faded and the colour drained from my cheeks as I realised that she wasn't pulling my leg.

'The bill is correct, Mrs Gunn. That is the cost of the treatment.'

It was her turn to go pale. '£250? £250?' She slumped lifelessly into the chair and for a moment I thought she had fainted.

'That's ridiculous, utterly ridiculous. I can't believe it,' she whined feebly. 'I thought it would cost between twenty five and thirty pounds.'

'It's a gold denture, Mrs Gunn. You'd get more than that for it if you melted it down and sold it as scrap. There's a lot of gold in it and gold is expensive.

'It isn't solid gold, is it?'

'Well, no it isn't. Solid gold would be much too soft.'

I cursed the fact that I hadn't quoted her properly in the first place and had wrongly assumed that she would know how much to expect.

'How many carats then?' she demanded beginning to look angry.

'About fifteen or sixteen I suppose but you can't really compare it with sixteen carat jewellery. The denture alloy is more expensive because it contains other precious metals such as platinum and silver. These other metals make the alloy harder and make it suitable for use as a denture base material.'

'Expensive is hardly the word for it. Extortionate, I would say.'

Having recovered from the initial shock she began to work herself up into a frenzy.

'What on earth am I going to do? Mr Gunn will go mad when he hears about it. What am I going to do? I don't know what I am going to do.' She burst into tears and started howling so loudly that her husband, who was downstairs in the waiting room heard her and came running up to see what was wrong.

'Look at this bill, Gerald. Look what Mr Derwent is trying to charge me for my treatment.'

Mr Gunn snatched the bill from his wife and winced noticeably as he read the total amount. 'Is this National Health?' he asked.

'No of course not,' I replied indignantly, 'the National Health service can't provide gold dentures.'

'Gold? Why did you make a gold one?'

'Because your wife asked for a gold one.'

'She never said anything to me about gold.'

'I had no idea it would be as expensive as that,' pleaded Mrs Gunn bursting into tears again. 'What will we do, Gerald?'

'Goodness knows,' replied Mr Gunn looking annoyed and worried at the same time. 'The only thing we can do is to use the money we were saving for our trip to America.'

'Does that mean we can't go?' sobbed Mrs Gunn.

'Not this year anyway. It's your fault, Ena. You're always ordering things without finding out how much they cost first. Perhaps you'll be more careful in future.

'I have been so looking forward to going to America. I need a holiday. I have to get away.'

'You've only yourself to blame. I still don't understand why you were stupid enough to ask for a gold denture.'

'Mr Derwent said it was the best and I wanted the best. You don't understand what it is like to have to wear a denture; you've got perfect teeth. It isn't very nice but as I have no choice but to wear one you can't blame me for wanting the best type.'

'Well, Mr Derwent would say it's the best, wouldn't he? He could see the pounds mounting up and you stupid enough to pay for it. Let's have a look at this wonderful denture then.'

Mrs Gunn drew back her lips but was hardly in the mood to give him a smile.

'No, take it out and let me have a proper look at it.'

Mrs Gunn extracted it from her mouth and handed it to her husband who examined it critically from all angles.

'Sheer extravagance,' he mumbled. 'Surely it could have been made from something cheaper. Wait a minute, though. If it's gold, why isn't it hallmarked? How do we know it isn't just plated?'

'I have never heard of a denture being hallmarked before,' I commented. In actual fact it had never occurred to me that anyone would want their dentures hallmarked.

'I want proof that it's really gold.' Mr Gunn handed the denture back to me. 'Get it hallmarked and then I'll consider paying for it. Come along, Ena, Mr Derwent can get in touch with us when he has done as I have asked.'

Mrs Gunn reluctantly picked up her old denture and put it in her mouth. 'Please do as he asks as quickly as you can, Mr Derwent. The new denture looks and feels so much better than this one.'

CHAPTER TWENTY

'Have you any idea how to get something hallmarked, Spencer?' I asked, desperate to try and salvage what nearly turned out to be a complete and utter disaster yesterday.

'Well, I have never done it before but I imagine you have to take it or send it to one of the Assay offices. What is it you want hallmarked?'

'Mrs Gunn's gold denture. Her husband says he won't pay for it until I get it hallmarked. They nearly had a fit when they got my bill for £250. They thought it was going to cost between £25 and £30.'

Spencer laughed out loud. 'Slight difference, but they should have realised that a gold denture was going to cost much more than that. There's a hell of a lot of gold in it, you can tell that by the weight. Surely they didn't really think that it would only cost £30?'

'Apparently they did. It was my fault, I should have quoted her properly for it in the first place.'

'Well yes I suppose so, but, it sounds as though she wouldn't have had a gold one if she had known it would be that expensive. They haven't said they won't pay for it, have they?'

'No, not exactly, but it has to be hallmarked first.'

'If I were you I would phone one of the Assay offices. I think they are only situated in the large cities, so there isn't one round here. I think London would be the nearest. Ring them up and ask them what you have to do. I'd get on to it right away if I were you; the sooner you get it done the sooner we get the money.'

'Do they have to cut off some of the metal to analyse it?'

'I have no idea, Justin.'

'It isn't going to do the denture much good if they have cut a piece off it for analysis. How they are going to stamp the hallmark onto it? The metal is very hard and it will take a lot of force to put their mark on it. I'm worried they might distort it in the process, and then it won't fit.'

'Justin, you are asking me questions I can't answer. You will have to make some enquiries.'

'Yes, I'll phone them some time this morning. Perhaps Beryl would find the telephone number for me. I have to go out in a moment. I'm going to St Margaret's Nursing Home. I'll phone when I get back.'

'What are you doing at St Margaret's?'

'I'm making a set of new dentures for one of the inmates. He couldn't get here because he is ninety two years old. So if the mountain won't come to Muhammad, Muhammad must go to the mountain. I have taken some impressions and, to save on the number of visits I will have to make, I did a sort of bite record at the same time.'

'A sort of bite record,' scoffed Spencer. 'I'll bet you anything it isn't accurate. I've often tried it myself and it never works. I don't think it pays to try to and cut corners. The bite will be wrong and you will have to go back again to put it right, so you won't save any time in the long run.'

'You are probably right but I thought it was worth a try. I had to soften some wax under the hot tap to take the bite, which wasn't easy so that reduces the chances of success still further. Do we have a spirit lamp or something similar I could take with me so that I can heat a wax knife in a flame?'

'Yes, I've got a spirit lamp somewhere, I will go and find it for you.'

As he left the surgery he passed Beryl who was on her way in to see me.

'Justin, Major Hetherington-Smythe has turned up downstairs.' She began. 'He's got the wrong day; he should have come tomorrow, but he said that as he is only here for a quick check to see how he is healing after his extractions surely you could fit him in this morning. I think you had better do something with him because there are quite a lot of people in the waiting room and he is telling them all that you nearly killed him last week. He's describing in graphic detail how you tore his gums to pieces, and that he thinks you should have sewn him up but wouldn't. He isn't doing your reputation any good at all.'

'I really ought to be going to St Margaret's Nursing Home, but I suppose I had better see him. Will you ask him to come straight up?'

Unfortunately the telephone rang at that moment so Beryl had to go and answer it. I decided that I had better fetch the Major myself. As I went down the stairs to the waiting room I could hear him say, 'Mr Derwent damned near killed me. Damned near killed me. He's nothing but a butcher.'

'Ah, Major Hetherington-Smythe,' I announced cheerily as I burst into the waiting room. 'Exaggerating again, I see. You are going to frighten these people off with such tales. They are probably wondering why you have risked coming back to see me again if I gave you such a hard time of it last week.'

'I'm only here because all you are going to do today is to check me out. You wouldn't see me for dust if I thought you were actually going to do some treatment. I couldn't go through that again. Damn near killed me.'

'Well let's go upstairs and I'll take a look.'

The Major's gums were healing very nicely, as I had expected. There wasn't really a problem. As far as I was concerned, the extractions had been straightforward and if he hadn't gone home and rinsed his mouth all day afterwards, he wouldn't have suffered excessive bleeding. I had arranged this follow up appointment just to put his mind at rest.

'Everything is fine, Major, and the gums are healing very well.'

'Thank God for that. I'll be off then and hope that I don't see you again for a very long time.'

'I would suggest you have a check-up in six months' time, then if something is going wrong we can catch it early and avoid the sort of situation you got into last time.'

'All right, Derwent, I take your point but I'll think about it in six months' time. Don't call me, I'll call you. Good day.'

After the Major had left I gathered together the things I needed to take with me to the nursing home. Domiciliary visits, as we called them, were a new experience to me and I didn't find it easy to remember everything I might want. Consequently I usually found that when I got there I had forgotten something. Spencer had stressed the importance of forward planning and suggested making a list but so far it hadn't worked well. One of the problems was that usually things were thrown into a bag at the last minute because of shortage of time. Today was no different thanks to the Major turning up unexpectedly.

'Here's the spirit lamp,' said Spencer. 'I've filled it with meths.'

It wasn't a very sophisticated piece of equipment, merely a glass lamp with a brass wick holder in the top, but hopefully it would do the job. Melvyn, the technician had set up some teeth in wax for me to try in the patient's mouth. They looked like complete dentures, but the bases were wax instead of plastic. He had used the bite record I had given to him to decide where to put the teeth and I hoped that the information had enabled him to set them in the right place. Spencer was sure they wouldn't be.

I enjoyed going to see patients at their homes, in hospital or in nursing homes. I was beginning to realise that one of the least enjoyable aspects of general practice dentistry was the fact that nearly all of it was spent confined to one room. It was a pleasant change, therefore, to be able to get into my car and drive off somewhere once in a while.

I felt quite important as I rang the doorbell at the nursing home carrying the leather Gladstone bag that Spencer had lent me.

'Good morning, I'm the dentist to see Mr Laidlaw,' I announced.

I was escorted along a maze of corridors, up a flight of stairs and along more corridors until I finally arrived at Mr Laidlaw's room.

Nursing homes were, to me, depressing places. They were usually similar to miniature hospitals inasmuch as the décor was very plain and usually quite tatty, and trolleys and wheelchairs adorned the corridors. The most striking feature, however, was that every nursing home I had been in seemed to have the same smell which was a curious mix of antiseptic, the smell you often find in the houses of old people, and the smell of cooking. The latter was not, however, the type of food smell you would encounter in a restaurant or hotel; it was more like school dinners.

'Hello, Mr Laidlaw, and how are you today?'

'Mustn't grumble, Mr Derwent. I'm not as young as I used to be, so I have to accept that I won't be as active as I was thirty years ago.'

I thought to myself, 'it's incredible to think that thirty years ago he would still have been over twice the age I am now. Looked at that way, life didn't seem quite so short; but then not everyone lives to be ninety two.'

'What are you going to do to me today then, Mr Derwent?'

'Nothing unpleasant, I assure you. I have got some dentures made of wax. I want to try them in to see if they fit, and to check that the teeth are in the right place.'

I took them out of my bag and placed them on the table. 'The teeth themselves aren't wax; they are the actual teeth I have chosen for you, but they are set in wax so that I can move them around easily if we need to.'

Mr Laidlaw removed his old dentures from his mouth and I slipped in the wax set. It was immediately apparent that Spencer was right; the teeth weren't in the right place, as they didn't meet properly when Mr Laidlaw bit together.

'I'm pleased with the appearance, Mr Laidlaw, they look good but I'm afraid we haven't quite got the bite right. The teeth don't come together properly so you wouldn't be able to eat very well with them.'

'That's no good then, Mr Derwent. I don't care what they look like – nobody will be looking at me at my age – but I've got to be able to eat with them, otherwise there isn't much point in having them.'

'Don't worry, Mr Laidlaw. As I said, the teeth are set in wax so I can move them, I'll just light my spirit lamp, soften the wax and reposition the back teeth so that they meet properly.'

The heat from Spencer's little lamp was quite intense and I had no difficulty heating up my knife to remove some of the teeth from the wax base. I removed all the lower back teeth from the right side and placed them on the table, then I set about melting the wax so that I could set the teeth into the new position. I had been working away for a few minutes when I suddenly became aware of an alarm bell sounding. 'Can you hear that bell, Mr Laidlaw? Do you know what it is?'

'I can't hear anything.'

'There's definitely a bell ringing. It sounds like an alarm of some sort.'

I wasn't kept wondering for much longer. A well-built nurse pushing a wheelchair opened the door and shouted 'fire alarm. Get outside immediately and assemble in the car park at the rear. I'll get Mr Laidlaw out.'

Mr Laidlaw was unceremoniously bundled into the wheelchair and propelled along the corridor at high speed by the buxom nurse whilst I followed on behind. When we arrived at the car park it was full of old people in wheelchairs. The staff had been very efficient in responding to the alarm and getting everyone outside. Many of the old people were very frail, some of them would have been bedridden, so it was all the more remarkable that they had been moved so quickly. There were just two nurses in attendance in the car park whilst all the other members of staff continued the evacuation process.

'Where's the fire?' I asked one of the nurses.

'We don't know yet. If the alarm goes off, the first priority is to get everyone outside, then we look for the fire unless it is obvious where it is. There is such a sensitive alarm system in the building that it will respond very quickly, hopefully before a fire has time to become established. It could even be a false alarm.'

'It's a big place. If you can't see a fire or smoke anywhere it could take a long time to locate it,' I remarked, thinking of all those corridors and rooms.

'The alarm system has zones so we can tell which part of the building is affected. That narrows it down to about half a dozen rooms, so if we still can't see the fire we carry out a thorough search of the area until we find a cause.'

'So you don't immediately call the fire brigade?'

'We used to, but we had so many false alarms; often it would be one of the patients having a crafty smoke that set off the alarm, so now we only call the fire brigade if someone has seen flames or serious smoke. No-one has seen anything so far this morning so we haven't called the fire brigade yet.'

'In which part of the building do you think it is?'

'It's somewhere in the east wing according to the control panel, that means rooms 46 to 52.'

'My room is 49,' said Mr Laidlaw through toothless gums. He was thrown into the wheelchair so quickly he wasn't even allowed time to put his dentures back in. 'So, the fire must be in one of the rooms next to, or very close to mine. To think we were so close to it. I must say the staff are very efficient in responding to the fire alarm. I didn't even hear it.'

'Are you warm enough, Mr Laidlaw?' said the nurse. 'I've got some blankets here if you want one.'

'I'm fine,' replied the old man, 'the excitement's keeping me warm. It isn't often we get this sort of entertainment. What do you think is happening now? I still can't see any fire.'

'Matron will be investigating the east wing together with the porter and a couple of other nurses, I should think,' said the nurse. 'If they find a small fire they will put it out with the fire extinguishers. If it's too big for that, they will summon the fire brigade. Oh, hang on, here they come now. They don't look in any hurry so I suspect they have either dealt with it, or it was a false alarm.'

'Thank goodness for that,' I sighed with relief. 'It would be terrible if fire ripped through the building.'

As the matron walked towards us I could see she was carrying a glass container. It didn't take long before I realised it was my, or rather Spencer's, spirit lamp. She held it up as she approached and looked straight at me.

'Is this yours?' she demanded.

'Er, yes, it is,' I confessed.

'Well, this is what set off the fire alarm.'

'I am terribly sorry,' I said, beside myself with embarrassment. 'I had no idea that your fire alarm was so sensitive. It never occurred to me for a moment that my spirit lamp would set it off.'

'You might have got away with it, except for the fact that your lamp was on the table in the centre of the room and the heat detector is on the ceiling directly above it,' explained the matron looking more than a little put out by the whole affair. The expression on her face left me in no doubt that she thought I had behaved rather stupidly and caused the entire nursing home a considerable amount of inconvenience.

Only Mr Laidlaw found the whole thing amusing.

'Ho, ho, ho,' he chuckled revealing his lack of teeth 'you naughty boy, Mr Derwent. Matron will probably give you a good spanking for what you've done.'

This remark sparked off guffaws of laughter from other staff members and those inmates who were sufficiently *compos mentis* to appreciate the joke. It also effectively augmented my embarrassment.

'Everyone back inside,' ordered the matron, handing the spirit lamp back to me.

'I haven't finished using it yet, Matron. Do you think it will be all right if I move it away from the heat detector? I don't want to set the alarm off again.'

'Well, at least we'll know what's causing it this time if it goes off again straightaway.'

Mr Laidlaw was taken back to his room in the wheelchair and I followed. As soon as he had been returned to his armchair, I set up the spirit lamp on the windowsill as far away from the heat detector as I could get it. I listened carefully but, thankfully, this time the alarm did not go off and I was able to reposition the teeth on Mr Laidlaw's dentures. I kept trying them in, and then I moved the teeth a little more until I was satisfied they were in exactly the right place.

'That looks better, Mr Laidlaw. They now meet at both sides when you close together. How do they feel to you?'

'All right, I think. I shall have a better idea when I've eaten my lunch with them.'

'Ah, I'm afraid you won't be able to do that today. The teeth are only set in wax; if you try eating with them the teeth will fall off. You will have to wait until the dentures are finished before you can eat with them.'

'When will that be, Mr Derwent?'

'Well, I know you said that you weren't worried about the appearance, but your family might be. After all, they will be the ones looking at your teeth. What I propose to do is to leave these wax dentures with you so that you can pop them in your mouth next time your family visit you. Then we can be sure that they are happy with the look of them.'

'Is that really necessary?'

'Yes I think it is, Mr Laidlaw. You see, once the dentures are completely finished, they can't easily be altered. At the moment, with the teeth set in wax, we can make adjustments. It is far better to make sure that everything is absolutely right before we finish them.'

'Well, if you say so, Mr Derwent, but I would like them as soon as possible. My son and his wife will be coming to see me over the weekend; they are the only ones who need to look at them.'

'Fine. Then I will come and see you again early next week and if everyone is happy with them I can get the dentures finished. Now remember, you must not try to eat with them.'

'I understand, Mr Derwent. I shall take great care of them, don't worry. I shall look forward to seeing you next week. Oh and by the way, try not to set any more alarms off on your way out; matron is not at all pleased with you as it is.'

There was a glint in his eye as he spoke and I thought what a wonderful old man he was, considering his age. Although he was a bit unsteady on his feet; mentally he was as bright as a button.

As I drove back to the surgery my thoughts turned to Mrs Gunn's denture. I hoped that Beryl would have found the telephone number of the London Assay office.

'What a nuisance,' I thought. 'If only I had quoted Mrs Gunn for the denture before I made it.' It occurred to me, however, that even if I had told her the cost before I made the denture, Mr Gunn would probably still have insisted on it being hallmarked.

Much to my surprise, Mrs Gunn was waiting for me when I got back to the surgery.

'Mr Derwent, can I have a word with you please?'

'Certainly, Mrs Gunn, come up to my surgery. As a matter of fact, I was just about to phone the London Assay office to try and arrange to have your denture hallmarked.'

'So you haven't sent it away?'

'No, not yet. I am still trying to sort it out.'

'Oh, thank goodness for that. I came round here hoping I would catch you before you sent it away. I've got the money here to settle your bill. It's my money and Mr Gunn doesn't know anything about it. For some time now I have been putting a little bit away to spend on myself. I have no idea what I was intending to do with it. I suppose I just thought it would be nice to have a little money set aside in case of emergency. It seems to me that Mr Gunn is making an unnecessary fuss about getting this denture hallmarked. As far as I am concerned, it felt and looked really good and I would like to have it without further delay, so I am here to pay for it and take it away if that's all right with you.'

'Why yes, of course, Mrs Gunn.' I made no attempt to hide my delight.

'I shan't say anything to Mr Gunn. I don't want him to know that I have saved up some money. He won't notice that I am wearing a new denture and in a couple of weeks' time, he will have forgotten everything about it.'

'You're sure he won't keep chasing me up to see if I've got it hallmarked and to find out why I haven't been in touch?'

'No, he won't. He doesn't take much interest in me or my affairs; he is too wrapped up in his own world. He'll forget about it completely.'

'I hope you're right, Mrs Gunn, but in any case, you are my patient, not him. If you come to me with the money for your new denture, I can hardly refuse to give it to you, can I? Here it is. Do you want to pop it in now?'

'Most certainly, Mr Derwent.'

Mrs Gunn slid the new denture into her mouth with all the skill and dexterity of an experienced denture wearer. 'That feels very comfortable.'

'That's good, Mrs Gunn. See how you get on when you try eating with it and if you have any problems at all don't hesitate to contact me immediately.'

'Yes, I will and thank you so much for all you have done for me. I am pleased I decided to have a gold denture.'

'It has been a pleasure, Mrs Gunn, and if I don't see you before, don't forget to come to have everything checked in six months' time.'

'You had better send me a reminder or I am likely to forget. Oh, by the way, how is your new nurse getting on? Sandra's her name, isn't it?'

'I'm afraid that didn't work out. She decided that dental nursing wasn't for her.'

'That's a shame. She seemed a nice girl, but a bit lacking in confidence. Never mind I am sure you will find someone suitable.'

'I hope so, Mrs Gunn, I do hope so, but it isn't easy to find the right person.'

'Well, good luck with the search and goodbye, Mr Derwent.'

CHAPTER TWENTY-ONE

I was now beginning to understand what the Dean of the dental school had meant when he told me that newly qualified dentists entering general practice can quickly become overwhelmed by financial commitments. I already had a bank loan for my car and, in spite of the fact that I was relatively well paid for someone of my age, my overdraft was steadily increasing. I had bought some new clothes, I liked eating out at good restaurants and I had also spent quite a lot on furniture and other items for the cottage I was renting. My latest display of extravagance was the acquisition of a good camera. I had always wanted one ever since I had taken some photographs with an old box camera as a child. Photography fascinated me and I could see that there was a good chance that it could develop into a serious hobby. If it did, this would no doubt result in considerable financial outlay in obtaining all the other items of equipment necessary to pursue the hobby.

I hadn't taken Tom Cox's advice about speaking to the members of the Luccombury Camera Club with regards to the type of camera I ought to buy; I was too impatient for that. On the next Saturday morning, I went along to the nearest camera shop and chose one I liked the look of. I knew that I wanted a 35 mm single lens reflex camera because I had seen other people using that type, but in actual fact my knowledge of them was very limited. I was prepared to accept the advice of the shop assistant who seemed to know what he was talking about. Whether his advice was governed by an attempt to choose the most suitable camera for me or by a desire to make as much profit as possible I shall never know, nor did it really matter. I came out of the shop clutching a piece of equipment with which I was delighted and which would, I felt sure, provide me with a great deal of enjoyment.

It seemed quite complicated but I welcomed the challenge of unravelling its mysteries and I studied the book of instructions from cover to cover. After about two hours, I felt I knew how to use the camera so I loaded it with film and went out. In the first flush of enthusiasm I photographed everything. Perhaps when the novelty had worn off I would learn to be more selective with my subject matter, but at the moment I was trigger-happy.

From my cottage I walked towards the nearby hills and woodland and reached a high vantage point overlooking the village. For the most part it had been a dull day but as I was approaching the top of the hill a break in the clouds allowed a yellow sunlight to cast long shadows over the landscape. It was breathtakingly beautiful; just the sort of scene one encounters from time to time when out walking but never, it seems, when one has a camera to hand. Today I did have a camera and thought that it was a tremendous stroke of luck that such a photographic opportunity should present itself to me on my very first day of camera ownership.

I was so excited I was worried that I might be shaking and not holding the camera still enough but I took some deep breaths and steadied myself down. I looked at the film counter which showed that I had already taken thirty two shots, so I had only four left, but that should be enough. In any case, I felt sure that someone had told me that very often you can get one or two extra frames on a film.

I took some time to compose the subject carefully, but I was aware that the light might fail at any moment so I had to be fairly quick. I exposed the last four frames varying the composition each time. The film continued to wind on and I got four bonus shots before the sun suddenly went in, bringing my opportunity to capture a photographic masterpiece to an end. I was amazed when I realised that I had got forty frames on the roll of film. One, or possibly two extra frames, was all I had expected; four extra frames seemed like extreme generosity on the part of the film manufacturer.

I wound the film back into the canister and removed it from the camera. Unfortunately I only had the one roll of film so I wouldn't be able to take any more photographs unless I could get some more film from the local chemist. I decided that I might try later, but as the weather had turned very dull again and it was now beginning to rain there didn't seem much point. Also, I was aware that the weather forecast for the next day was very bad. In the meantime, however, I was thrilled with the possibility that I might have taken a really spectacular photograph, one that I would be proud to show at the camera club if I were to join. It might even be good enough to enter in a photographic competition. My imagination went into overdrive as I walked back to my cottage.

As soon as I got back I telephoned Tom Cox.

'Hello, Justin.'

'I am phoning to tell you that I bought a new camera this morning, and this afternoon when the sun broke through the clouds I was up on the hills overlooking Luccombury and I think I might have taken a really stunning photograph.'

'The light was wonderful for a few minutes. I thought at the time that if you were in the right place you might get a really good shot. Unfortunately, I was working on my car so I missed the opportunity. I always say that photography is all about being in the right place at the right time. If you can grab one of these fleeting moments you might, just might, have a winner. I hope you were successful.'

'I really phoned up to ask if I could take you up on your offer to go with you to the Luccombury Camera Club.'

'Sure, they meet on Monday evenings at seven thirty. If you want to go on Monday, I'll pick you up at your cottage just after seven.'

'That would be great.'

'Until Monday, then.'

The weather forecast for Sunday turned out to be perfectly accurate and totally unsuitable for taking photographs. I spent the day reading photographic books and magazines in front of an open fire in my cottage. It was a very lazy but thoroughly enjoyable way to spend a wet day.

All day Monday I thought of little else but my camera and photography in general. At lunchtime I took my film to the local chemist to get it developed and I made an effort to get home early in order to have a quick meal and get ready for the Camera Club. I had just finished eating when the phone rang. It was Tom.

'Justin, I know we had arranged to go to the Camera Club, but something else much more interesting has turned up. I have been doing some research on local organisations that might be a good source of female talent for unattached young men like you and me. I've discovered this club, which is for the young, single, divorced and separated. It's called The Bankks Club, spelt with a double 'k' for some reason. During the summer they play tennis then go on to a pub afterwards. Apparently the women greatly outnumber the men – it sounds ideal. Tonight they are playing tennis at Winsome Park, and I said that you and I would be very happy to join them.'

I didn't share Tom's enthusiasm. I particularly wanted to go to the Camera Club, and the idea of playing tennis struck a note of panic within me. I immediately thought that they would probably all be accomplished players. I had never been very good, and what's more I hadn't played at all since I left school. Why was every young man I met in Luccombury obsessed with the idea of hunting for a girlfriend? Richard Darcy certainly was, and now it appeared that Tom had the same idea. I didn't really care whether I had a girlfriend or not. If one came along, all well and good – in fact very good – but I wasn't all that interested in going out to look for one specifically. Playing tennis certainly didn't seem a very good way for me to make a good impression on a girl.

'I thought you and Carolyn were together,' I replied, desperately trying to find a way to pour cold water on Tom's plans for the evening.

'Oh, Lyn and I have known each other for many years and I think the world of her, but she knows that I get restless and feel the need to have my freedom from time to time. She has come to realise that she is unlikely to get a long-term commitment from me and she understands. I am still very much on the market when it comes to women and I know you are unattached. Anyway, I will pick you up just after seven, as arranged, but bring your tennis racquet instead of your camera.'

'I'm afraid I don't have a tennis racquet,' I replied feebly. I knew as I said it that it wouldn't deter Tom and I was right.

'Don't worry, I think I have a spare one lying around somewhere. I'll look it out for you. See you later, must dash now.'

'Damn,' I thought. I had been looking forward to going to the Camera Club and I was not very keen on playing tennis at the best of times – certainly not with complete strangers who were probably a hundred times better than me at the game.

I always thought that one would meet members of the opposite sex during one's normal daily life and, from time to time, meet someone with whom one wanted to strike up a relationship. I never thought that it would be necessary to go out hunting for them like wild boar. I wasn't keen on picking up girls in pubs like Richard Darcy, and I didn't think that getting to know someone over a game of tennis was a good idea either.

I just couldn't understand why Tom wasn't happy with Carolyn as his girlfriend. From what I had seen of her she was perfectly lovely, both in appearance and personality. He would find it extremely difficult to find someone better. I had no experience of clubs for single, divorced and separated people, but I had a strong suspicion that it would consist mainly of divorcees who had been severely traumatised emotionally by their past experiences and, as a result, now carried huge psychological hang-ups. Perhaps this was an excessively cynical point of view.

When Tom arrived, I was horrified to see how sporty he looked. He was wearing tennis shorts and a white sleeveless sweater over a white shirt.

'I don't have any tennis gear, I'm afraid,' I announced, feeling slightly awkward in my blue shirt and grey trousers.

'Don't worry, I'm sure it won't matter,' he replied nonchalantly.

'Do you play tennis often?' I asked him, hoping that he wouldn't be too expert.

'About three times a week, and I usually have a lesson as well.'

The words landed like lead and made me more convinced that I should have found an excuse to get out of going. However, it was too late for that now. I was well and truly committed.

When we arrived at the courts some people were already playing. On one court a match of mixed doubles was already under way. They all looked extremely professional in their white tennis outfits and the standard of play appeared to me to be incredibly high. I was worried that I would be made to look a complete idiot if I had to play with someone even half as good.

A tall, athletic young man came over to greet us.

'Welcome to the Bankks Club, glad you could come,' he shouted. 'I'm Colin.'

We shook hands and introduced ourselves to him.

'You may be wondering where the name Bankks came from. It is the initials of the names of the people who founded the club five years ago. Bridget, Andrew, Neil, Karen, Keith and Susan. It was established as a social club for people to make friends, but tennis has always featured strongly in the club's activities and it is so popular we play virtually every week during the summer. Come and meet some of the other members.'

There were about twenty five people there altogether and, as Tom had predicted, the women outnumbered the men by about two to one.

'How's your tennis, then?' asked Colin. 'Not that it matters whether you are an expert or a complete beginner; everyone is welcome.'

That made me feel a bit better but I was anxious to make my position clear from the start and so I returned promptly, 'definitely a beginner.'

'That's fine,' said Colin, 'but I'll guarantee that if you keep coming to the club you'll be absolutely amazed how quickly you will improve. We have several beginners. so you won't feel out of your depth. How about you, Tom?'

'I've been playing for some time but I still have a lot to learn.'

'Haven't we all? Okay, you go to court number 3 and I'll fix you up with some others. Justin, you come with me.

He took me to one of the courts where three other members were obviously waiting for a fourth person to join them so they could start their game.

'Hi folks, this is Justin,' announced Colin, 'Justin, meet Annette, Sarah and David. Have a good game.'

David was quite tall and slim and didn't look half as athletic as Colin. Annette was petite with short dark hair and I couldn't help noticing she had nice legs. Sarah was taller, slimmer and had medium length blonde hair tied back. Unlike the other two, who were in conventional tennis outfits, she wore a light blue tracksuit.

'I'll play with you,' said Sarah to me.

'Okay' agreed David. 'Come on Annette, let's give them a good thrashing.'

I needn't have had any inhibitions about my tennis because we were all of much the same standard. The game wasn't taken very seriously and, although David and Annette did win, it could hardly be described as 'a thrashing'. I thought that we would probably change partners and play another game, but Sarah proposed that we went to the pub for a drink ahead of all the other members, including Tom, who were still playing with great vigour and enthusiasm.

I had in fact quite enjoyed the game once I had overcome my initial apprehension and I felt sure that the exercise would be good for me. However, I didn't raise any objections to Sarah's suggestion, and Annette and David also seemed perfectly willing to go along with it. We put our racquets away and soon we were sipping drinks in the lounge bar of the Black Dog.

'Half an hour's tennis is enough for me after a busy day at work,' said Sarah who looked as if she was really enjoying her drink. 'My job is quite energetic enough anyway.'

'What do you do?'

'I'm a physio. I work at the Chiropractic clinic at Venwood. Do you know it?'

'I'm afraid not,' I replied, 'I have only been in the area a short time.'

'So have I,' said Sarah. 'I came from Kent two months ago. My mother wanted to come here because she said the weather was milder and she has a brother who lives just outside Luccombury. What do you do for a living?'

'I'm a dentist.'

'Really? You don't look like a dentist.'

'Why not? What's a dentist supposed to look like?'

'You look, well … too nice, really. I thought you had to be a bit hard with a cruel streak to be a dentist.'

'Don't be fooled by appearances. I love inflicting pain, particularly on defenceless old ladies. I'm as hard as nails really.'

'I don't believe you,' laughed Sarah. 'What made you come to the Bankks Club?'

'I came with Tom; he arranged it. I hadn't heard of the club until this evening. We were supposed to be going to the Luccombury Camera Club but Tom decided he preferred to come here. I just got dragged along.'

'Are you keen on photography?'

'Yes, I think so. I mean. I've only just bought a camera, but photography has always interested me and I thought the Camera Club would be a good way to learn more about it. To be honest, I didn't really want to come here. I was disappointed when he decided not to take me to the Camera Club.'

'And are you still disappointed?'

'No. I quite enjoyed playing tennis and everyone here seems very friendly.'

'Well I'm glad you came.'

At that moment, some of the other members of the club came into the bar. Tom followed shortly after. His eyes were twinkling. 'You didn't stick the tennis for long.' He smiled as he looked long and hard at Sarah.

'Long enough I think, Tom. When you haven't played for about six years, it isn't wise to overdo it first time out. Do you want a drink?'

'Thanks, I'll have a pint of bitter.'

Sarah's glass was empty so I picked it up and went to the bar. When I returned with the drinks, Tom had taken my seat next to Sarah and was chatting away to her, so I put the drinks down in front of them and found another vacant seat next to Annette and David.

I discovered that Annette worked for a bank and David was a schoolteacher. They had both joined the Bankks Club within the past few months and seemed to be enjoying the tennis, though they admitted that the main attraction was the friendships they had established. I wasn't sure whether they were in fact going out together, or whether they just met on Bankks Club nights.

I chatted with them, and other members of the club came over from time to time to join in the conversation. The evening passed very quickly and soon it was closing time. Tom, who had spent the entire evening talking to Sarah said to me, 'Come on, Justin, I'll take you home now.'

I wished everyone goodnight and soon Tom and I were in his car heading back to my cottage.

'I think Sarah fancies you,' he declared suddenly.

'Whatever makes you say that?' I was more than a little taken aback by his statement.

'She asked a lot of questions about you. I told her that I had only just met you myself so I couldn't provide the answers. I hope you don't think I muscled in on you by pinching your seat and sitting with her, but I must admit I like the look of her. I reckon that, up to a point, all's fair in love and war. I wouldn't deliberately set out to steal another chap's girlfriend, but as you had only known her for about an hour I didn't think you had any special claim to her, so I thought I'd give it a try. Unfortunately she didn't want to know. I invited her out but she politely refused. I think she would go out with you, though.'

'It never occurred to me for a moment that she might be interested in me. We just had a game of tennis together with David and Annette, and then we chatted for a short time until you arrived.'

'I think you made quite an impression on her. I notice these things and it isn't very often I'm wrong. She's an attractive girl – tall, slim and blonde – what more do you want? I would certainly be interested but, as I said, I didn't get anywhere with her. How do you feel about it? Are you interested?'

'I don't know, I hadn't really thought about it.'

'Well I think it's worth giving some thought to it. The only problem is that she and her mother are going back to Kent at the weekend to sort out some business. They won't be back for six weeks so you will have plenty of time to think about how you want to play it when she gets back.'

I wasn't sure whether or not I wanted to enter into a relationship with Sarah, but I know that I felt some disappointment when I heard that she was going to be away for six weeks. Perhaps I was just flattered to think that she might be interested in me.

'Did you enjoy this evening?'

'Yes I did. Thanks for taking me, Tom. It was a good idea of yours, but I would have been happy to go to the Camera Club.'

'I know, and we will go and check it out but I have heard that the average age of the Camera Club members is about seventy. I thought there were some very attractive women at the Bankks Club and it would have been a shame to miss the opportunity to meet them. There could be some exciting possibilities there and we haven't even scratched the surface yet, though you seem to have got off to a good start.'

'I don't know about that, Tom. I can't believe what you've said about Sarah.'

'I'm telling you, Justin, I am rarely wrong about these things. Anyway do you want to continue to go to the Bankks Club?'

'Yes, I would like to go again.'

'It looks as if the Camera Club will have go on the back burner for the time being. It's a pity both clubs meet on Monday evenings.'

CHAPTER TWENTY-TWO

'How's the weight chart looking?' I called out to Spencer as I passed his surgery door. I could see he was staring hard at the graph, having presumably just entered today's weight on the chart.

'Not too bad,' he replied somewhat unconvincingly.

I went over to his desk to look at it though I got the distinct impression he would have preferred me not to.

'My weight is coming down but perhaps not as quickly as I had hoped.'

The graph showing his progress over the past few weeks oscillated up and down and close examination showed that there was a miniscule downward progression. He was, in fact, about half a stone lighter today than six weeks ago.

'How much did you say you wanted to lose?'

'I need to lose another stone and a half before I go on holiday which is in six weeks' time.'

'It seems then that you are going to have to try harder, bearing in mind that you've only lost half a stone in the past six weeks.'

'I know. I can't understand why I haven't lost more. I'm not eating much; in fact, I'm starving hungry for most of the time. It's very depressing, Justin. People who don't have a weight problem like yourself can't begin to appreciate what we fatties go through.'

'It is true that I can eat whatever I want to but in actual fact I don't eat a lot of sweets, cakes or biscuits. I don't like them very much. I have noticed that you have a lot of sugar in your tea and coffee and I often see you munching something during the day. I think you have a very sweet tooth and I also think that if you were to add it all up, you would probably find that you eat much more in a day than I do.'

'I couldn't bear the idea of unsweetened coffee, though I suppose I could get some artificial sweeteners. I try not to pick at things during the day but if I find sweets lying around I tend to eat them and Beryl is always bringing biscuits here. I don't realise I'm doing it much of the time, I suppose it's comfort eating. From now on I will try a lot harder. If you see me eating anything during the day tell me about it and stop me doing it.'

'I'll try if that's what you want.'

'I'm afraid it's necessary if I'm to reach my target weight by the time I go on holiday. Anyway, changing the subject, I have good news for you about your nurse. I have interviewed the German girl and I have to say that I think she will be very good. She is bright, quick to learn and looks efficient. The main drawback is that she is younger than I would have liked. As you know, I wanted an old battle-axe who would keep you and the patients in check. I think an older nurse is better able to exert her authority with patients, which is often to the dentist's advantage. Unfortunately it has been very difficult to find anyone to fill the vacancy, so I couldn't be too choosy. I am sure you will be delighted with her because she is very attractive. Her name is Ingrid and she is coming to meet you this afternoon.'

'That's great news, Spencer. I'm looking forward to meeting her. She sounds like just the sort of girl I would have chosen for myself if you had afforded me the opportunity.'

'Steady on now, Justin, don't get over excited about it. The other reason I wanted someone older for you is that you are young, unattached, and with a twinkle in your eye. Working day in, day out, with a pretty young nurse could lead to other things. I don't think it is a good idea to have a personal relationship with one's nurse. It's all right as long as nothing goes wrong with the relationship. but if it does it then becomes very difficult to work together.'

'Yes, I can see that Spencer, but I'm getting a bit tired of everyone thinking I can't wait to get off with some woman or other. Richard Darcy seems to think that that's the only thing in life that matters – his whole life revolves around looking for a woman, and Tom Cox was trying to get me off with someone at the Club we went to on Monday evening. Now you're on about me getting involved with my nurse!'

'All right, all right, I just thought I'd make the point.'

'Anyway, wasn't Daphne your nurse?'

'No, she was my father's nurse. You can go off with Beryl if you want to, but keep your hands off your own nurse.'

'Right, I'll remember that. What time is Ingrid coming this afternoon?'

'We didn't fix a time. I just said come to the surgery sometime during the afternoon. What have you got lined up for this morning?'

'First I'm seeing John Pendleton for an extraction. Do you know him?'

'I don't think so. I can't remember seeing him.'

'No he doesn't come very often – only when he's in pain. He should do really because he's got terrible teeth. He's got decay everywhere. I'm extracting one of his upper premolars which is completely shot to pieces, and I shall be most surprised if I don't have to extract some of his others as well. Nice enough chap, but he just hates dentistry.'

'Patients like that are difficult. They don't seek regular treatment because they don't like coming, and then when they are finally driven here by pain we have to subject them to loads of fillings and often extractions so the whole thing turns out to be a thoroughly unpleasant experience for them, which only increases their fear of dental treatment.'

'I suspect his diet, like yours, consists of far too much sugar. I think I will question him about it and see if I can give him some advice on cutting down on the things that rot his teeth.'

'If you ask me, that's a complete waste of time. In my experience it is very difficult, if not impossible, to persuade people to change their habits. You can talk to them until you are blue in the face and they might change for a short time, but they always slip back into their old ways eventually.'

'That's a cynical view, Spencer. Gum specialists maintain that nearly all gum disease can be cured by teaching patients better oral hygiene and getting them on to the right diet. Are you saying that they are never successful because patients can't be motivated?'

'I think they enjoy short-term success. One of the reasons why patients might follow their advice for a time is the fact that they pay huge amounts of money for the specialist treatment. You are hardly likely to pay someone hundreds of pounds for his advice and then immediately ignore it, are you? However, when the memory of the cost of the treatment has faded they slip back into their old ways. In my opinion, only a tiny proportion of patients are permanently cured of gum disease, in spite of what the specialists say. They would obviously like us to believe they achieve miracle cures but I am not convinced.'

'It's an interesting theory.'

'Well, it's just my opinion but I can name a number of patients for whom it is true. What are you doing after John Pendleton?'

'I'm going to see Mr Laidlaw again at St Margaret's.'

'Haven't you finished his dentures yet?'

'No. You were right about the makeshift bite record being inaccurate. I reset the teeth last time at the nursing home, as well as causing the place to be evacuated by triggering the fire alarm. I left the wax try-in with him so that he could let his family have a look. If they are happy with the appearance, I can send it off to Melvyn to get it finished. I think Mr Pendleton has arrived now, so I had better get on.'

John Pendleton was in his early forties but looked considerably older. He stood an inch or two over five feet tall and was almost as wide. The bold checked shirt he was wearing and the fact that the supermarket bag he was carrying almost trailed along the floor as he walked, along with his peculiar rolling motion, emphasised his lack of height. He found climbing the stairs from the waiting room very hard work and by the time he reached my surgery he was breathless for some minutes. I gave him some time to compose himself before addressing him.

'I'm very concerned about the amount of tooth decay you have in your mouth, Mr Pendleton. Would you say that your diet consists of a lot of sugary things?'

'I eat too many sweets, Mr Derwent, I know I do. You see, I work in a sweet factory. The policy of the management is to allow the workers to eat as many sweets as they like whilst they are working. Most people gorge themselves in the first couple of weeks, then they get sick of the sight of them and rarely eat any more. This is what the management bank on and it nearly always works. Unfortunately, in my case it didn't. I eat just as many now as I did on my first day.'

'Dear oh dear, Mr Pendleton, no wonder your teeth are decaying. Have you tried to stop eating them?'

'I try every day and sometimes I might manage to go through most of the morning without eating any, but come the afternoon my willpower fails me. The only way I could stop eating them would be to find another job. It's really strange because I never eat them when I'm at home, nor when I'm on holiday, but when I'm at work and they are all passing before me on the conveyor belt I can't stop myself picking up the odd one or two. I suppose one would say I'm addicted to them in a funny sort of way.'

'Yes, I suppose so,' I agreed. 'It's a real problem for you, Mr Pendleton, but as far as your teeth are concerned if you don't stop eating sweets you won't have any of them left soon.'

'I really will try to stop, or at least cut down, Mr Derwent, but I've been trying to do that for so long now don't hold out much hope that I'll succeed.'

There didn't seem to be much point in lecturing him any further. The cause of his dental problems had been isolated and now it was up to him. 'I'll do what I can to save as many of your teeth as possible, but I'm afraid the broken one up there will have to come out.'

'I know there is nothing you can do with that one. I am dreading having it out though, Mr Derwent. I'm a real coward when it comes to dentists. I feel so nervous about it.'

'Don't worry, it'll be fine. We'll get rid of that one today, then we'll make some appointments to try and fill as many of the others as we can.'

'I am most grateful to you. I hate dental treatment, but I also dreaded coming because I was embarrassed about the state of my teeth. I thought you might tell me off.'

'I'm here to help you, Mr Pendleton, not to tell you off.'

'You are very kind, Mr Derwent. I thought that when I saw you two weeks ago. I am so grateful I have brought you a little present.'

He picked up the supermarket bag and handed it to me.

'You shouldn't have done that,' I said as I took it from him. It was quite heavy and when I opened it I saw that it was absolutely full of liquorice allsorts.

'Er, thank you, Mr Pendleton, I am very grateful to you. I suppose these are the sort of sweets you eat on a daily basis.'

'Just one of the many. We make lots of different sweets: toffees, spearmint chews, jelly babies, fruit pastilles, you name it, we probably make it.'

'I shall share this bag of sweets with the other members of the practice, but it will last us ages and ages. I mustn't let my patients see me eating them, as it wouldn't set a very good example.'

'No, I suppose not. Anyway, I hope you will enjoy them, Mr Derwent. Now can we get this tooth out? I'd like to get it over and done with as soon as possible.'

'Yes, of course.'

I rubbed some local anaesthetic paste on to his gum and waited two or three minutes for it to go numb before I injected the anaesthetic solution. As the injection site was near the front of the mouth, the paste didn't numb Mr Pendleton's throat, so I didn't encounter the problem I had experienced with Major Hetherington-Smythe when he was convinced he was choking. I slid the needle in slowly and gently and injected the solution quite painlessly.

'Would you like to rinse out your mouth now, Mr Pendleton?'

He did as I suggested and then placed the mouthwash glass back on the holder and got up out of the dental chair.

'Brilliant, Mr Derwent, I didn't feel a thing. I just didn't know it was coming out. You're a marvel.'

'That was just the injection. The tooth isn't out yet.'

'Isn't it? I thought it was. I rinsed out blood.'

'That was just a little bit of blood from the injection. Sit down again.'

His elation drained away before me and a look of terror took over. Reluctantly he sank back into the chair.

I was aware that extracting teeth from bull-necked young men could sometimes be very difficult; their teeth were often very firmly fixed. In this particular case, it didn't help that the tooth was badly broken down and there wasn't anything solid to get hold of. There was a good chance that as soon as I tried to grip it with the forceps it would shatter. Mr Pendleton's confidence, what little he had, would no doubt shatter at the same time.

I placed the beaks of the forceps around the tooth and pushed hard upwards to get as far down the root as possible. As soon as I tightened my grip, the tooth shot out of the forceps and out of Mr Pendleton's mouth with amazing velocity. The roots were tapered and, just like when you squeeze on a slippery cone with finger and thumb and the cone shoots away from you, the tooth did the same thing when the beaks of the forceps squeezed it.

'By golly, Mr Derwent, that positively shot out. How did you do that? Usually there's a whole lot of pulling and tugging. That was very clever and I didn't feel anything.'

'I can't promise to do that every time I take out a tooth. It was the shape of the root that caused it to come out like that. I must admit it was quite a surprise to me too. I was expecting it to be much more difficult.'

'Can I go now?'

'Yes you can but don't forget to make another appointment. Go and see Beryl in the office and she will arrange it for you.'

'Right, Mr Derwent. I can come anytime you want me to. I don't have any trouble getting time off work, so it can be whenever suits you. My time is your time.'

'Great. I'll see you again soon then, Mr Pendleton. Goodbye.'

I was very relieved that Mr Pendleton's tooth had come out so easily. I had feared that it was going to take a long time and might be very unpleasant for him. Luck had been on my side on this occasion.

I turned my attention to getting things ready for my visit to St Margaret's Nursing Home and Mr Laidlaw. I packed Spencer's Gladstone bag with everything I might possibly need and, as the extraction on Mr Pendleton had been accomplished much quicker than anticipated, I had some time to kill. I took the opportunity to catch up with some paperwork and a quarter of an hour later I was ready to set off.

As I came out of my surgery I could hear Mr Pendleton's voice in the office, so I went to see why he was still here.

Beryl was looking quite exasperated. 'Justin, I am finding it impossible to arrange Mr Pendleton's next appointment. He wants to know if you work on Saturday afternoons. He can't manage any of the times I've offered him.'

'I don't work on Saturday afternoons. Anyway, you said you could come any time,' I said to him.

'I know, and usually I can, but it just so happens that I can't come on the days I've been offered.'

'Well, you tell us when you can come.'

Mr Pendleton thumbed backwards and forwards through his diary. 'What about seven o'clock on Monday the 27th?'

'My last appointment is at five o'clock.'

'I meant seven o'clock in the morning, then I could come before I go to work.'

'I'm sorry, the first appointment is at nine o'clock. You said that you didn't have any trouble getting time off work.'

'I don't normally, but I've just remembered that we are going to be short-staffed for the next four weeks so I can't really be spared.'

'So what you are saying, in effect, is that for the next four weeks you won't be able to get here between nine and five during the week, nor on a Saturday morning?'

'I'm afraid so. I'm sorry.'

'In that case we'll have to make your next appointment in five weeks' time.'

'But that's a long way off. Don't I need to come sooner?'

'If you can't get here during normal office hours then that's the best we can do. You can always phone up if you find there is a day you could come; we'll see if we can fit you in.'

Mr Pendleton realised that this was my final offer and gracefully withdrew, though he was obviously not totally happy about it.

'We'll see you in five weeks then, and thank you for the liquorice allsorts,'

'Oh yes, you're welcome. Until the next time, then. Goodbye.'

'What's this about liquorice allsorts?' Beryl asked as soon as Mr Pendleton was out of the room.

'Mr Pendleton has given me this huge bag. I don't really know what to do with them. I don't often eat sweets. I'll leave them here for now. Help yourself to them if you like.'

'Thank you, Justin, and thank you Mr Pendleton, but I don't often eat sweets either. I'll think about who we can give them to. I'm sure someone would be glad of them.'

'Good idea, Beryl. In the meantime, I'm off to see Mr Laidlaw at St Margaret's.'

CHAPTER TWENTY-THREE

The familiar smell of the nursing home greeted me as I opened the door of the main entrance. Olfactory evidence of cooking was particularly strong today and I felt sure it was a stew of some sort. It was not at all inviting and if I had been invited to stay to lunch I would have declined.

I no longer had to introduce myself; the episode with the fire alarm meant that I was now well known to all the members of staff. They didn't even escort me to Mr Laidlaw's room anymore.

'You know where to go, Mr Derwent?'

'Yes thank you.'

'Let us know if you need anything.'

What had originally seemed a long and tortuous route to room 49 was now perfectly straightforward for me.

'Good morning, Mr Laidlaw,' I called out cheerily, 'and how are you today?'

'I'm well, thank you, Mr Derwent. How are you?'

'I'm fine, thank you. It's a lovely morning isn't it? The sun is streaming in through your window.'

'I know. I should be on the beach today, not stuck in here. There will be lots of young ladies in their bikinis on a day like this.'

'Now, now, Mr Laidlaw, think of your blood pressure. In any case, I doubt if there will be that many. The weather looks nice but it's quite cold.'

'It's still early in the year, isn't it? Perhaps I'll stay where I am today then.'

'A wise decision if I may say so. What did your family think about your dentures. Did they like them?'

Mr Laidlaw suddenly became evasive. 'Er yes, I think so, but it was a bit difficult for them.'

'What do you mean?'

'It was a bit difficult for them to give an opinion.'

'Why? Did you put them in and let them have a look?'

'There wasn't much point, really.'

'Why not, Mr Laidlaw? That was the whole point of the exercise.'

'I know but I had a slight accident.'

'What exactly do you mean?'

'Well, on Thursday I was given a lovely lamb chop for dinner. It looked absolutely delicious with mint sauce and redcurrant jelly. I did so want to enjoy it, but my old dentures were making my mouth sore and so I thought that I would give your dentures a try. I know you said I shouldn't eat with them because the teeth were only in wax, but I thought it would be all right if I ate gently.'

'And what happened? Don't tell me – the teeth came off.'

'They did I'm afraid, Mr Derwent. They're over there.'

I went over to where the dentures were sitting on a shelf. I could see immediately that not a single tooth remained in the wax bases.

'Not a tooth left in there, Mr Laidlaw. Every one of them has come out.'

'I'm afraid so, Mr Derwent. I'm sorry.'

'So this happened on Thursday, before your family had chance to look at them?'

'That's right. That's why they weren't able to say what they thought of them.'

'Have you got the teeth?'

'No, I don't know where they went.'

'You didn't swallow them did you, Mr Laidlaw?'

'I don't know. I don't think I did. I'm sure I spat them out. When I felt something hard in my mouth I thought it was a piece of bone from the lamb chop. Then I felt another and another, and I realised it was the teeth off the dentures. I spat them on to my plate and I thought I'd better save them for you.'

'So where are they now?'

'Oh dear, I'm so sorry, Mr Derwent. I took them off my plate and put them into a piece of tissue. Unfortunately I forgot about them and must have used the tissue to wipe my mouth or something. Later, I suddenly remembered about the teeth and couldn't find the tissue. I eventually found it in the waste paper bin, but there was no sign of the teeth.'

'What, none of them?'

'No, I couldn't find any.'

'Did you empty the waste bin right out to look?'

'I went through it.'

Quite automatically my eyes started to scan the floor in the vain hope of finding at least some of the teeth. Immediately I spotted something small and white by the table leg – sure enough it was an artificial molar. I picked it up and continued my search of the floor. On hands and knees I scoured the beige carpet and after three or four minutes I had recovered no less than ten of the twenty eight teeth.

'How often do they hoover your carpet?'

'Every day.'

'And empty your waste bin?'

'Every day.'

It was now Tuesday, so on that basis the vacuum cleaner had been over the carpet probably four times since the teeth came off the dentures.

'It's lucky for us they don't seem to do a very thorough job of hoovering, Mr Laidlaw. Let's see how thoroughly they empty the waste bin.'

I tipped out the contents on to a newspaper and found another eight teeth in the bottom.

'Only ten more to go.'

Unfortunately, further searching failed to recover any more, and after ten minutes or so I abandoned the attempt.

'I'm afraid this puts us back quite a long way, Mr Laidlaw. I am going to have to order up some more teeth to replace the missing ones, and then we have to set them into the wax once more and try them in your mouth to check that we have got them in the right place. We then come up against the problem of letting your family have a look at them, which is where we were last week.'

'Can't you just put the teeth back and finish the dentures without all that messing about? I shall be dead by the time I get them at this rate. In any case they are bound to be better than my old dentures – they must be forty years old.'

'It's a bit risky to cut corners like that, but I can understand you wanting to have the dentures as soon as possible. I'll see what I can do. I'll be in touch as soon as I am in a position for us to move on.'

I left the nursing home and decided to call in at the chemist on my way back to the surgery to see if my film had been developed. I was really excited about it as I felt sure I had photographed something very special. Everything had been just right and there could be no possible reason why I had not got a winning photograph.

I handed in my slip to the assistant who seemed to take forever to locate the envelope with my name on it; such was my impatience.

'There seems to have been a problem with this one, Mr Derwent. They haven't printed any photographs – they developed the film but didn't print it for some reason. Let me see what they say – they usually put a note inside.'

I didn't know what to say. 'A problem? How could there be? What sort of problem?' My first thought was that something had gone wrong at the laboratory. I would be furious if they had messed up the film. There were important pictures on it.

'Here's the note,' said the assistant. 'It appears that the film was blank – nothing on it at all. Either the camera shutter isn't opening or the film didn't go through the camera. The most likely explanation, they think, is that the film wasn't wound on to the take up spool so it stayed in the cassette.'

I couldn't believe it. The disappointment was overwhelming. Surely that couldn't be right. I paid the assistant the nominal sum for developing the film and came out of the shop crestfallen. I took the film from the envelope just to check but it was as they said, completely blank from start to finish.

'How could that have happened?' I wondered. My conclusion after I had accepted that the mistake must have been mine was that in my inexperience, I had failed to wind the film far enough on to the take up spool before closing the camera. The recollection that the film had apparently not reached the end after forty exposures came back to me. That should have set the alarm bells ringing. How stupid of me not to realise that it isn't possible to get forty frames on a thirty-six exposure film. I was bitterly disappointed that my prize-winning photograph had not materialised but I hoped that I would learn from this incident and not make the same mistake again in the future. I would put the episode behind me now and not dwell on it any longer.

As I made my way to the surgery, my thoughts turned back to Mr Laidlaw and how this latest little problem with his dentures could have been avoided. I was well aware that I was still new to the problems of general practice dentistry and I wanted to try and learn from this sort of situation in order to try and avoid the same thing happening again. But it seemed to me that perhaps one had to accept that there was no way to prevent it. I had felt it necessary to leave the dentures with Mr Laidlaw so that he could show them to his family and I had told him that he must not eat with them, or I thought I had. Perhaps I hadn't given enough emphasis to the fact that if he did try to eat with them they would be completely ruined and we would be more or less back to square one. Was it now wise to try and put the teeth back into what I thought was the right position and then finish the dentures without checking and without letting Mr Laidlaw's family look at them first? I was under pressure from Mr Laidlaw to get the dentures finished as quickly as possible but if I succumbed to this pressure would I be letting myself in for further problems. What if the teeth didn't go back into the right position and as a result, Mr Laidlaw couldn't wear them, or what if Mr Laidlaw's family said they didn't like them. I really didn't know what to do for the best and decided to seek Spencer's advice.

On entering the surgery I went straight to the office. Spencer came out just as I arrived. I spoke to him but received only a muffled grunt in reply. His cheeks were puffed out and he appeared to have his mouth full of something. I was slightly puzzled by his behaviour especially as he seemed anxious to get away from me. Beryl quickly let me know what he was up to.

'He hasn't stopped eating those liquorice allsorts since you left.'

I looked at the supermarket bag, which was considerably less full than when Mr Pendleton had given it to me.

'Has anyone else had any?' I asked Beryl.

'No. Spencer is the only one. He's been coming in here every few minutes and filling his mouth with as many as he could cram in.'

'He's eaten loads. So much for his diet! Did you say anything to him?'

'It's not up to me to try and stop him.'

'He told me I had to stop him eating sweets, cakes, biscuits and the like. He'll never lose weight for his holiday at this rate.'

'He's had the weight chart out again, has he? Before every holiday it's the same but I'm convinced he never actually achieves his target. I think he fiddles the chart half the time.'

'I'm going to have a word with him for his own good.'

By the time I confronted him in his surgery, Spencer had emptied his mouth and was sitting at his desk like a naughty schoolboy.

'I can't resist liquorice allsorts, Justin. I haven't had many really.'

'You said I had to stop you eating things like that, so just one is one too many. It seems to me that you have eaten a great pile of them. It doesn't matter to me how fat you become. I'm simply trying to save you from yourself because you asked me to stop you eating fattening things.'

'I know and thank you for your concern. I won't eat any more of them.'

CHAPTER TWENTY-FOUR

I didn't see much of Spencer for the rest of the day because soon after lunch Ingrid arrived, and I spent a lot of time talking to her and teaching her about dentistry in general. There was a great deal to tell someone who had no previous experience of dental nursing.

Beryl told me that Spencer had continued to sneak into the office and fill his mouth with liquorice allsorts whenever he felt he could get away with it. She hadn't actually castigated him about it, believing that it was nothing to do with her, so she hadn't made him feel guilty as I would have done. He took advantage of the fact that I was occupied with Ingrid and, therefore, out of his way.

On this particular day he left the surgery at about four o'clock because he had to attend a meeting of the Luccombury Agricultural Society, of which he was chairman for the current year. He was very proud to have had this office bestowed upon him and spent a lot of time engaged in the affairs of the society.

The meeting was held in the Luccombury Village Hall, which was situated about half a mile away from the surgery and on this occasion, as the weather was quite pleasant, he chose to walk rather than take his Rolls Royce. He liked to arrive early to set out his papers before him and organise his thoughts before too many people arrived to distract him. He prided himself on handling meetings effectively, making sure that all speakers kept to the point by intervening wherever necessary to keep them on track. He had chaired numerous other committees over the years and he believed he was quite good at it. Indeed, many other members of the society also thought that he was a firstclass chairman.

The Village Hall was not large, and although it was quite old, it was soundly built of stone and well maintained. Its layout was very simple consisting of just a main hall and a well-equipped kitchen, and at some stage, a small walk-in cupboard at one end of the main hall had been converted to a makeshift cloakroom. It was customary for the committee to sit around a long table, which was created by putting together a number of small fold-up tables at the cloakroom end of the room. This particular spot was chosen because there was more natural light from the windows and there were more heaters at this end of the room. Spencer quickly set up the table and chairs and took up his position at the head of it. Soon other members of the committee began to arrive.

Shortly after opening the meeting, Spencer became aware that his stomach was beginning to rumble rather noisily. In fact it became so loud that he felt sure that other members of the committee would be able to hear it. Some of them noticed that he was shuffling around uneasily as he went through the matters arising from the minutes of the previous meeting, and they may have heard his stomach rumbling, but no one passed comment.

The truth of the matter was that the rumblings of Spencer's stomach were becoming louder and more violent. He was also aware now that the mild abdominal pain he had experienced at the start of the meeting was rapidly gathering intensity.

The treasurer's report seemed to go on and on and Spencer wondered how there could be so much to report when the society's bank balance was a mere £86. The secretary's report was interminable and it is doubtful if Spencer heard a word of it. His ability to concentrate on the meeting was failing him by the minute because the abdominal discomfort he was experiencing was now becoming intolerable. All he wanted was to announce the date of the next meeting and bring this one to a close but there were still a number of items on the agenda which had not yet been dealt with.

His shuffling became more pronounced and by now it had been noticed by all the committee members, though most of them did not feel it was appropriate to mention it, even though they must have wondered what was the matter with him.

Normally he was so well organised and efficient, so totally in control and composed. The secretary, who had been aware for some time that Spencer's attention was diverted for some reason, could stand it no longer and asked him outright if there was something wrong. Spencer assured him that there wasn't, but as his obvious unease did not abate, no one was convinced.

By now peristaltic waves were almost lifting Spencer out of his chair, his face was purple and beads of perspiration were dripping from his brow. The pain within him followed a cyclical pattern, building up to a crescendo then slowly subsiding to a slightly less excruciating level. The relief was mercifully welcome but unfortunately the moments of respite were short lived and were replaced by ferocious bouts of griping colic, which progressively increased in strength with each new attack.

Should he make a desperate but undignified sortie to the cloakroom where he felt sure he could secure almost instant release from this agonising and disabling condition, which at the present time was destroying his ability even to think straight? For a moment he thought he would – he would have to, he had no choice – then suddenly as well as fighting off the pain and pressing urgency, he fought off the temptation to take this course of action because he knew it would be cringingly embarrassing for him.

One glance at the cloakroom door brought home to him how flimsy and ill-fitting it was; the degree of privacy afforded by it was minimal in the extreme. What made it worse was that the two most supercilious members of the committee, Air Commodore Barrington and Lady Harcourt, were sitting barely three feet away from it. The installation of the cloakroom had been very much a compromise in a building which had no real facility for such a commodity. Its real purpose was to cater for the elderly, cut short due to their intake of diuretic tablets. However, it was woefully inadequate to deal with an acute gastrointestinal episode of the sort of magnitude afflicting Spencer that evening.

He took some deep breaths and shuffled some more in his seat in the vain hope that a change of position might bring even a particle of relief from his anguish. As the peristaltic movements gathered momentum once again he went through the mental torment over whether he should try to sit it out to the end of the meeting or submit to the degradation of making a lightning dash to the cloakroom. He was frantic to end his torture but, at the same time, phrenetic to maintain the decorum expected of him, both as a professional person and chairman of the committee.

The meeting continued without any involvement from him, other than an occasional interjection. What little input he had was designed primarily to speed the meeting along and he almost made it to the end. He dutifully asked if there was any other business, praying that there wouldn't be. Sadly for him, one of the members produced a list of issues she wished to bring to the attention of the committee. Spencer's determination to see the meeting through to the end was instantly shattered by the startling inevitability that it was likely to continue for a further indefinite period. At the same time a blast of pain swept through him like a tsunami, shaking his very being to the core. For a moment he felt as if he would literally explode.

This was breaking point and resulted in discretion intervening and ousting his resolve to remain in his chair until the end of the meeting. He finally accepted that this was no longer merely a pressing need; it was the end of the road and unless common sense prevailed, he would suffer the ultimate humiliation there and then in the presence of the rest of the committee without even a flimsy door to hide his shame.

'You will have to excuse me,' he blurted out as he made a frenzied sprint past the astounded committee members. He almost wrenched the feeble cloakroom door off its hinges in his desperation to get to the other side of it.

Any doubts that Spencer may have had about the effectiveness of liquorice as a laxative were well and truly laid to rest that evening.

CHAPTER TWENTY-FIVE

Who on earth could be phoning me at this time on a Sunday morning? It wasn't even half past seven and the weather was foul. It was raining hard and blowing a gale as well.

'Hi, Justin, it's Tom Cox here. Sorry to disturb you so early, but I wondered what you were doing today.'

'I haven't got anything planned and, looking at the weather, there isn't much one can do outside. I was hoping it might clear up later so that I could go out with my camera, but I'm not sure where at the moment.'

'I wondered if you would do me a favour.'

'I will if I can. What is it?'

'Would you be prepared to come out for the day and make up a foursome? I don't know if you met a girl called Vanessa at the Bankks Club last Monday? I don't think you did. She wasn't there for long but I spoke to her briefly and seemed to get on well with her, so I phoned her up and asked her out. She said that she would come as long as Annette could come as well, and suggested that I get someone else to make up a foursome. I wondered if you might like to join us.'

'I thought Annette was going out with David? Didn't he want to go with her?'

'No, they aren't going out together. They just like to play tennis together because they are both about the same standard. In fact, it seems that David has his sights on someone else. I'm only asking you to make up the party. There are no strings attached.'

'Does Annette know that you are asking me?'

'I'm not sure. I told Vanessa that I might ask you, but I don't know if she has mentioned it to Annette. In any case it doesn't matter. I told you, there are no strings attached.'

'Where are you going? The weather is absolutely terrible.'

'I know it is. The forecast isn't that brilliant either, though one forecast I heard said better weather was coming in this afternoon. I had originally thought we might go for a drive somewhere, have a walk in the country and call in for a pub lunch. The weather seems to have put paid to that idea. I don't suppose anybody wants to go walking in this and, to be honest, I'm a bit worried about my boat; it's blowing about a force nine here. It's moored at Arne and my worry is that other people often moor alongside and don't always tie on securely. In a gale like this if another boat is moving about alongside they can both take a battering, so I really wanted to go and check that it's all right. It's not a very exciting way to spend the day, but you might be interested to see the boat and we can have a cup of tea on board and a game of cards or something, and then if the weather clears we can move on. I haven't put the idea to the girls yet, but as I said, in this weather there isn't a lot you can do.'

'I can see that you need to go and check on your boat. I would be happy to join you, as long as it's all right with the girls.'

'I'm sure it will be. That's great, thanks, Justin. So why don't you drive to my house about ten o'clock and then we'll go and pick the girls up in my car? Oh, and bring your camera.'

'I'll see you later, then.'

I wasn't sure whether I wanted to go or not. I didn't mind doing Tom a favour, though I still couldn't understand why he felt it necessary to go running after girls when he had someone like Carolyn as a long-term friend. I didn't think I was being paired off with Annette; Tom had made it clear that I was being invited purely to make up the party. It would be interesting to see his boat, and there might be some opportunity to take photographs, which is what I really wanted to do.

I hadn't been to his house before and I wasn't sure what to expect. It was certainly in a secluded setting, up a long rough track and surrounded by trees. The nearest neighbour was about three hundred yards away. The house was relatively modern compared with most of the houses in the area and, although beautifully situated, did not have a lot of character. Tom heard my tyres on the gravel drive as I approached and came to the door to greet me.

'Welcome to Cox Towers,' he called out.

'You said it was out in the sticks. I can now see what you mean. It's a lovely setting.' I looked up to see the treetops bending alarmingly in the wind. There were several mature trees close enough to Tom's house to make an awful mess of it if they were to be uprooted and happened to fall in the wrong direction.

'Yes, I like it. Since I bought it I've spent more time away than I have here but I've decided that I'm here to stay now, at least for a while. I'm finished with sailing long distances. I shall use the boat to potter around the coast for the odd day or weekend, but I'm not interested in anything more than that right now. Unless, of course, I meet someone I want to sail off with. Frankly, I'm worried about the way the weather seems to be behaving these days. It seems much more unpredictable than it used to be, and you wouldn't want to be out on the high seas in these conditions.'

Tom led me inside. We entered through the back door straight into the kitchen, which was somewhat basic but functional. There was a strong nautical influence in that it was galley-style in its layout and the wall cupboards, which had been made by Tom, were more like the lockers on a boat than kitchen units. We went through to his sitting room, which was even more basic. What little furniture there was in there looked as if it had come from a jumble sale. A battered old sofa faced the open fireplace, which contained the remains of a log fire. Alongside it was an armchair of a completely different style and colour from the sofa. The only other items of furniture in the spacious room were a big old pine table, four odd wooden chairs and an oak bookcase. There was a tattered rug in front of the fireplace and the rest of the floor was covered with sheets of hardboard rather than carpet.

'As you can see,' said Tom, 'I haven't really got around to doing anything with this other than to make it more or less habitable.'

'It has great potential,' I replied enthusiastically. ' It's very spacious, and there is a wonderful view of the garden.'

'Yes, it could be very comfortable. I'm planning on improving it a bit now that I shall be living here. It will all get done in time. Anyway, let's go and meet the girls. I phoned Vanessa after speaking to you and explained that I ought to go and see that my boat is all right in this wind. She said she didn't mind at all and was looking forward to seeing it. Apparently Annette was quite excited to hear that you might be coming along.'

'Oh really?'

'Yes. Vanessa and Annette spoke to each other last night and Vanessa told her that I was arranging for someone else to join us to make up the party and that I thought of asking you. Annette said that she hoped you would come. Hang on, I'll just get my camera from out of the safe.'

The 'safe' turned out to be under a cushion on the sofa. I would have been most surprised if any determined burglar failed to find it. The house was so remote that when it was left unoccupied a burglar would have all the time in the world to search undisturbed for anything worth stealing. Tom, however, had left the house empty for long periods without any problems. Burglary in this part of the country must be less prevalent than in the north of England.

The rain was beating down harder than ever and we had to make a dash for Tom's car, which was parked at the front of the house. He never parked it in his garage because that was full of tools and yachting equipment.

When we arrived at Vanessa's house, the girls were waiting for us in the porch and immediately ran out to join us in the car. I said hello to Annette, and Tom introduced me to Vanessa. She was tall; in fact, I guessed that she might be slightly taller than Tom. Her figure was slim and athletic, and she had short brown hair and very dark eyes. Her smile was very attractive and came easily. It seemed to me that she had the sort of bubbly personality that appealed to Tom. He opened the conversation.

'I was hoping to take you on a rather special walk today. It's about five miles long, some of it through woodland and some of it with spectacular cliff top views over the sea. I discovered it quite by chance. Unfortunately, I'm afraid the good Lord overlooked my request for good weather. However, I am thankful I'm not out sailing.'

'According to the weather forecast I heard, the wind is expected to die down this afternoon and there might even be some sunshine' said Vanessa.

'Let's hope so.'

It took us about half an hour to drive to where Tom's boat was moored. I hadn't been there before and it looked an interesting part of the country. The river at this point was about fifty feet wide, and there were lots of small and medium sized yachts tied up there.

'That's mine there,' said Tom pointing to a very smart white and blue schooner, which was moored right up to the riverbank. Another boat of similar size was tied alongside it. The wind was still blowing fiercely and the boats were moving around quite a lot.

'We need to get some more ropes onto them,' called Tom as he jumped out of his car. I got out with him and awaited his instructions, but he didn't need any help. In no time at all he had secured both boats to his satisfaction.

' Okay everyone, you can go on board now.'

We went below and closed the hatch. The cabin was beautifully finished with lots of varnished wood, but it was unexpectedly cramped. It must have felt very small when out in the middle of the vast Atlantic Ocean.

'I'll put the kettle on,' said Tom.

Everything on board was in miniature. The kettle was tiny, the sink was tiny, and so was the hob, which apparently ran on paraffin. The fridge and cooker were diminutive versions of the appliances one would have in a normal kitchen.

'It's bobbing about quite a lot, isn't it?' remarked Annette who was sitting very close to me at one side of the small fold-down table.

'It's still blowing a good force eight, but I do think it looks a little bit brighter over those hills,' replied Tom optimistically.

'It doesn't look any brighter to me,' Vanessa remarked in a matter-of-fact tone of voice.

'When you go sailing, you always have to try and remain positive,' laughed Tom. 'I can remember when Carolyn and I were about five days out to sea in the Atlantic and a storm blew up. It wasn't quite as bad as this but still bad enough and we kept saying to each other "I think it is beginning to clear," or "I don't think it's blowing quite as hard now as it was half an hour ago". I suppose we were each trying to comfort the other because at the back of your mind you are thinking "if this gets much worse we could be in real trouble".'

'Frankly, Tom, I think you must be either very brave or mad to even consider sailing across the Atlantic in a boat as small as this,' I remarked.

'So do I,' agreed Annette.

'I think it's a jolly good way to get away from civilisation and all the little annoyances of daily routine for a while,' declared Vanessa.

'So you would be happy to come with me if I did the trip again, would you, Vanessa?'

'I might be.'

I was inclined to think that Vanessa's assessment of the present weather situation was more accurate than Tom's; the wind and rain didn't seem to be easing, and the boat was rocking about more than ever. Suddenly Annette stood up.

'I'm going to have to get off the boat, Tom. I'm no sailor, I'm afraid, and I shall be ill if I stay on here much longer.'

The movement of the boat had become more apparent to me when I saw that my tea was swilling around in the cup. I then noticed through the porthole that the distant skyline was going up and down and I had to admit that I wasn't enjoying watching it. Once I became aware of it for some reason I couldn't stop looking at it and I can remember wishing it would keep still.

'I'll go with Annette, Tom. We'll go and sit in the car,' I announced chivalrously.

'Are you sure you don't mind?'

'No, not at all.'

'I'm sorry to drag you away, Justin,' Annette said once we were safely in Tom's car.

'Don't be, Annette. I don't mind at all. In fact, to be honest, I think the movement of the boat was beginning to get to me. I'm no sailor either.'

'We wouldn't be any good crossing the Atlantic in it, would we?' she laughed.

'Good Lord, no. Seasickness is a terrible thing. Someone once said to me that for the first half hour you are afraid you are going to die, and after that you are afraid you aren't.'

'Yes, I think that just about sums it up. I'm really glad you joined the Bankks Club, Justin. I enjoyed playing tennis with you. Will you be going again next week?'

'Yes, I think so. I enjoyed playing tennis, though I'm not very good at it, but I do need the exercise.'

'I thought you played well, especially as you hadn't played for six years.'

'No, I have a long way to go before I can claim to be a good player.'

'It really doesn't matter how good or bad you are, as long as you enjoy it. I enjoy the company more than the tennis.'

'When did you join the club?'

'About six months ago, soon after I moved to Luccombury from London. I had to get away and try to make a new start in life. I'd been suffering from severe depression and I decided that I needed a complete change of surroundings, a new job and new friends.'

'It sounds a very drastic move. Has it worked out for you?'

'It is going to take time but I think it was the right thing to do and I am getting better slowly.'

'Did you come on your own?'

'Yes. My mother still lives in London and I go back to see her every other weekend, but she didn't want to move and I didn't feel I could force her. In fact, it's probably better that she didn't come. I need to make my own way.'

'Was there a particular reason for your depression?'

'Yes there was. It hurts me to talk about it.'

I could see that Annette was becoming upset and I felt that it would be best if I didn't pursue it any further.

'I'm sorry, Annette, I shouldn't have asked. We can change the subject if it upsets you.'

'You have such a kind face, Justin. I haven't told many people but I feel I can tell you. I was engaged to be married, the wedding was all arranged, it was to be quite a big occasion with over a hundred guests. Everything seemed perfect, the weather was warm and sunny, it promised to be a wonderful day, until …'

Annette paused and her eyes showed an inner sadness. 'Marc jilted me at the altar.'

Annette's last few words caused her great pain. She broke down in tears as she spoke and threw her arms around me, sobbing against my shoulder. Suddenly, I realised that Tom was standing by the car and he opened the door with a smile on his face.

'Hello, hello, so what are you two up to?' he began, misreading the situation. When he saw that Annette was crying he quickly changed his approach.

'Is there something wrong?'

'It's all right, Tom. Annette is a bit upset about something but she'll be fine in a minute. She just needed to talk about it.'

'I'm so sorry,' said Annette, drying her eyes. 'I shouldn't have burdened you with my troubles. Please forget I mentioned it.'

'Don't worry. I understand how you must feel and you were right to tell me if it helped you in any way.' Instinctively I took hold of her hand to comfort her and I soon got the impression that she was in no hurry for me to let go of it.

Tom and Vanessa got into the car.

'There isn't any real reason to stay here now,' said Tom. 'I think the wind is easing and I have made the boat secure so we can move on. I suggest we go and get some lunch. There's a lovely little pub about two miles from here.'

'Sounds like a good idea, Tom,' I replied. 'We liked your boat but I think it's fair to say that Annette and I preferred to admire it from the riverbank.'

'Definitely,' added Annette, who was now looking a bit more composed.

We had a very pleasant and leisurely lunch in the lounge bar of the pub in front of a log fire. Conversation was lively and we soon felt that we had all known each other for a long time and were quite relaxed together. Vanessa and Tom seemed to be getting on well and talked a lot about sailing. Tom was very happy to relate his maritime experiences, as well as his exploits during his stay in America. It made me feel that, by comparison, I had led a very narrow and unadventurous life, but if I were honest about it, I had no great desire to travel very far. I felt that the English countryside had an enormous amount to offer and I could be perfectly happy exploring the area around Luccombury. Foreign travel held little appeal for me. It was clear, however, that Vanessa had a great longing to see the world and that she derived great pleasure from asking Tom about some of the exotic places he had visited. After a couple of hours I was quite sure that if Tom invited her to sail off somewhere with him she would accept immediately. I wasn't sure whether it was because she liked him as a person, or whether it was simply the prospect of the adventure that was so alluring.

After lunch we drove down to the coast and were able to go for a brief stroll along the cliff tops. The weather had improved considerably but remained very breezy and showery, so none of us wanted to walk a long way. Annette stuck close to me most of the time and was quite happy when Tom and Vanessa became engrossed in conversation with each other and walked some distance in front or behind us. We got on well together and chatted about all sorts of things, from our school days to our favourite foods, our tastes in music and books we had read.

We were all quite windswept when we got back into Tom's car and when he suggested that we went back to his house to get the fire going and open a bottle of wine, we all thought it was an excellent idea.

Although there wasn't a lot of comfort in his sitting room, no-one minded in the slightest. Annette and Vanessa were quite content to sit on the floor soaking up the warmth of the fire whilst I played with Tom's camera. There hadn't been much opportunity to take photographs, though Tom had taken one or two of the girls on the cliff tops with the sea behind them. At the time, they complained about being photographed because they felt they were so dishevelled but Tom had done his best to convince them that they both looked stunning.

Vanessa was the first to notice that for the past twenty minutes or so, Tom had not been sitting with us but was pottering about in his kitchen. She got up and went out to see what he was doing.

'Just rustling us up a bite to eat,' came his reply. 'The sea air has made me hungry. I expect you are too.'

'It certainly smells good, Tom. What are you cooking?'

'Spaghetti Bolognese.'

Soon the four of us were tucking into Tom's culinary creation. Spaghetti Bolognese was not the sort of food I chose to eat very often but on this occasion, washed down with a very pleasant red wine, it tasted fantastic.

It had been a most enjoyable day even though we hadn't done very much. I was pleased that Spencer and Daphne had introduced me to Tom, and I could see that he and I could become very good friends. It was clear that through him I would get to meet lots of other nice people. The evening passed very quickly as we continued chatting away. Tom and Vanessa spent most of it sitting shoulder to shoulder on the floor, whilst Annette and I shared the sofa. None of us was anxious to break up the party but finally Vanessa declared that she ought to be making a move because she had an early start the next day.

We all piled back into Tom's car to drive the girls back home. There was no real need for me to go with them. I could have gone straight home in my car, but I wanted to enjoy the company for as long as possible. We said goodnight to them and Tom turned the car round to set off back to his house.

'It was a good day, Tom. Thank you for inviting me to join you.'

'Yes, I enjoyed it too.' He replied. 'I like the look of Vanessa. I think she could be a lot of fun. What do you think?'

'Yes, I think she's very nice, and attractive too. Are you going to ask her out again?'

'Yes, most definitely. I'll see if I can get her to come out with me on her own next time. How did you get on with Annette?'

' Alright, but I don't see anything more than friendship there.'

'Well, if you want my opinion you would be well away with her. I think she fancies you.'

'No. Whatever makes you say that? That business in the car wasn't anything. She just threw her arms around me because she was upset about something that happened to her not very long ago. I was just comforting her, that's all.'

'I wasn't referring to that. I realised that it must be something like that after the initial shock of seeing her in your arms.' He grinned cheekily at me as he spoke. 'No, I could tell she fancied you by the way she looked at you and was trying to get close to you all the time. Didn't you notice?'

'No, I didn't notice. You were telling me only the other day that Sarah fancied me.'

'Yes, I'm sure she does. What is wrong with you, Justin? You have all these gorgeous women swooning at your feet and you don't even notice?'

I couldn't really believe what Tom was telling me. Annette and I got on well together, but I can honestly say that I saw no more in it than that. Nor for that matter had I considered for one moment that Sarah might be interested in more than just friendship with me. His words set me thinking. Perhaps I ought to loosen up a bit and emerge from my shell. Both Tom and Richard Darcy were in no doubt at all that women were worth chasing. Perhaps I didn't realise what I was missing.

CHAPTER TWENTY-SIX

'Can I have a few words with you after surgery, please Spencer? I would like your advice on Mr Laidlaw's dentures.'

'Ah, Mr Laidlaw! So the saga continues. Sure, Justin, I should be finished by five thirty. Come down to the sitting room after your last patient. In fact, I wanted to speak to you. I am going up to London tomorrow for three days and so you will be left in sole charge here. I need to fill you in on one or two patients who might want to see you whilst I'm away.'

'Right, I'll meet up with you later then.'

Now that Ingrid was settling in to dental nursing, I was able to work much faster and more efficiently. I could see from my daybook that the result of this was that I was also earning more money, a fact that had not gone unnoticed by Spencer.

Ingrid was exceedingly bright and quick to learn. In fact, the point had now been reached where she was sometimes a step ahead of me. I would ask her to go and get something for me, only to find that she had anticipated my request and already had it in her hand waiting to pass it to me.

I had always believed that German people were well organised and efficient, and Ingrid certainly confirmed this. As an added bonus she was very good-looking with a kind, open face and lively hazel eyes. Her grasp of English was first class and it was rare for her to encounter a word with which she was not familiar. She spoke well and retained just enough of a German accent for it to be attractive. Her friendly and jovial manner endeared her immediately to the patients and I had to admit that, this time, Spencer had done well in his quest to find me a nurse. We worked well together and surgery life had improved considerably since she came onto the scene. She made it quite clear, however, that she considered British dentists, based presumably on what she had seen of Spencer and I, were very much the poor relations when compared with dentists in Germany.

'Dentists in Germany are so rich,' she said, her eyes widening. 'They only work two or three days a week and drive big expensive cars. You know, it costs a lot of money to get dental treatment. They charge four or five times as much as you for a crown.'

'People here think our fees are too high,' I replied. 'They have been spoilt by the National Health Service and expect their dental treatment to be free.'

'Yes I suppose so,' she conceded. 'But this surgery is so old-fashioned compared with the one I used to go to in Berlin. That was so streamlined with all the very latest equipment. The surgeries were very big with hidden lighting round the walls and kitchen type units for the instruments. There seemed to be lots of nurses and they all wore light blue trouser suits, whilst the dentists were in white suits.'

'I think some of the dental practices in London might be like that, but we are in rural Dorset and life moves more slowly out here.'

'Yes, I can see that, but I think Spencer is more behind the times than most, don't you? His equipment is so old. I have never seen a dental chair like his and it is so uncomfortable to sit in. His drill doesn't really work properly. It keeps shooting off the tubing whilst he is drilling.'

'Spencer's father bought the equipment many years ago and when it was made they didn't have high speed drills. They were invented much later and so Spencer carried out a modification himself to try to bring it up to date. I think he bought a second hand drill unit from somewhere and rigged it up to an old compressor from his workshop.'

'Well, it looks very crude and doesn't work very well either, and he still has the slow drill driven with string.'

'You mean the cord-driven drill?'

'Yes, that's it. They don't have them in Germany.'

'They probably did years ago. There aren't many of them left in this country. Modern dental units have small electric motors or small air motors for the slow speed drill. Spencer hasn't moved in that direction yet, but at least he has moved on from the foot engine.'

'The foot engine? What's that?'

'If you look in the cupboard under the stairs you will see a drill that is operated by treadling with the foot. It's what dentists used before electrically operated drills were invented.'

'Oh my goodness, Why has he still got it? He doesn't use it, does he?'

'Apparently he does from time to time when there is a power cut. It seems that the electricity supply can be unreliable around here; it often goes off if there are high winds or a thunderstorm. It hasn't happened since I came here, but last winter the power went off several times and Spencer was able to keep on working by using his foot engine.'

'Good heavens,' said Ingrid looking absolutely horrified. 'Have you ever used one, Justin?'

'No. I don't think I would be any good with it. It must be quite difficult to keep the drill steady in someone's mouth and treadle like mad with your foot at the same time.'

'What you need, Justin, is a nurse with big powerful thighs who can do the – how you say, *treadling*? – for you. I would have a go for you if you wanted me to but I'm not sure that I would be able to generate enough power; my thighs are probably not strong enough.'

'It's very kind of you to offer, Ingrid, but I hope the need won't arise. Anyway, your thighs look perfect to me just as they are.'

When Ingrid wasn't actually working in the surgery she frequently wore a mini-skirt, so I was able to speak with some knowledge on that particular subject. Unfortunately, Spencer happened to walk into my surgery at that moment and heard my last remark.

'What's all this about Ingrid's thighs, Justin? I trust you haven't forgotten our conversation about maintaining a professional relationship with one's nurse?'

'No I haven't, Spencer. We were talking about your foot engine and I said that I would find it difficult to drill and treadle at the same time. Ingrid said that if the need arose she would try to operate the treadle for me, but was concerned that her thighs weren't strong enough to be able to generate sufficient power.'

Spencer looked at me with some scepticism, but before he could say anything else Ingrid continued.

'I was saying that your surgery and equipment is – do you say *antiquated*? – compared with dental surgeries in Germany. Look at your X-ray machine; it's an absolute monster. At the dentist I used to go to in Germany, every surgery had its own X-ray machine and they were very small things mounted on the wall. I have noticed too that yours makes a funny noise every time you use it. I'm sure it shouldn't do that.'

Spencer suddenly became very defensive. 'There is absolutely nothing wrong with the X-ray machine. It works perfectly and I am confident it will continue to do so for many years to come. It is big, I admit that, but that is because it is solidly made, not like the modern machines which won't last five minutes. Now, haven't you two any patients to see?'

'Ingrid is just about to get the next one in for me.'

'Good. Well, I'll let you get on then.'

Spencer stomped out of my surgery bearing one of his more pompous expressions. I am sure he was well aware just how outdated his equipment looked to everybody, but he had nothing but contempt for modern dental equipment which he said was like modern cars – not built to last and the other point to consider was that whilst he was a complete spendthrift when it came to holidays or other treats for himself, he absolutely hated spending money on anything for the surgery.

Ingrid and I sailed through the afternoon without any problems and, as I said goodbye to her when she left to go home I thought once again what a great asset she would be for the practice. It did occur to me, however, that she was very capable and intelligent and might decide, as Anna had, that she could do something better with her life than dental nursing.

Spencer was already in his sitting room when I went downstairs at just after half past five,

'Come in and have a beer, Justin. Have you had a good day?'

'Yes, not too bad at all. I have managed to get through quite a lot of work today, as you will see from my daybook.'

'I have noticed that you are doing more work now that you have Ingrid to help you.'

'Yes, she is very good. She has learnt the job very quickly and is now a great help to me.'

'Well, I told you I would find you a good nurse, didn't I? I would have been happier if she hadn't been quite so young and attractive, but you can't have everything. You seem to work well together. In fact, you seem to be settling in very well here, Justin. how do you feel about it? are you happy?'

'Oh yes, I am enjoying general practice. I sometimes miss my university friends, but there is a lot going on here and I am beginning to make new friends now. It's certainly very nice not to be penniless for a change.'

'Dentistry has its compensations, but I sometimes think it is a strange sort of job.'

'Why do you say that?'

'It can be very narrow in that you are working in the same little room virtually all the time.'

'Except for the odd home visit.'

'Yes, but mostly in your own surgery. You can't really converse with people in the normal way, because if you are talking to them you aren't getting on with the job or they are too nervous to want to chat with you. You have little contact with other members of the profession so it is a fairly insular type of existence. That's why I think it is important to have lots of outside interests.'

'I suppose it is a funny sort of job if you analyse it. Many people seem to think it's odd that anyone would want to be a dentist.'

'Yes they do. I have discovered over the years that it is best not to tell strangers what you do for a living because they never fail to be completely fascinated. Their response is always the same and takes three phases. The first is disbelief that anyone would want to do a job which they see as being the infliction of pain on other human beings. They think there must be something very curious about you to make you want to do that. They then ask why it is that after their dentist has filled their mouth with equipment and his fingers so that they can't talk, he then starts to ask them questions. The third phase, and the one which is the hardest to tolerate, is the fact that, for some reason, they believe that you are longing to hear about the time a dentist had his foot on their chest trying to extract a tooth, or some other similarly harrowing experience suffered at the hands of a member of our profession.'

I laughed at Spencer's analysis of human behaviour in relation to dentists. I can't say that I had experienced this response exactly, but it was certainly true that people seemed to think you would be interested in their dental history.

'If anyone asks what I do for a living,' Spencer continued, 'I tell them I'm an interior decorator, which isn't too far from the truth. Anyway, what is it about Mr Laidlaw's dentures you want to ask me?'

'You know we had a disaster because he tried eating with the wax dentures and all the teeth fell off? Well, he is very anxious to get these dentures finished as soon as possible and wants me to press on with them. He says it isn't necessary to show his family before we finish them and I must admit the job is dragging on now and I would like to see the back of it. I haven't rechecked the bite since I put all the teeth back so it might not be quite right, but I can always grind it in afterwards, as long as it isn't too far out. The question is, do I risk going ahead and finish them or do I go back to square one?'

'Justin,' Spencer began in a distinctly paternal tone, 'just think what will happen if the bite is a long way out. You'll never be able to grind it in satisfactorily, which means that the dentures will be useless. And what if his family don't like them when they are finished? You'll have to start the whole job over again from the very beginning which, as well as being a financial disaster for you, won't do your reputation any good. You must remember always that it is a golden rule that we never allow the demands of patients and the pressures they often try to put us under to influence our clinical judgement. It doesn't matter what the patient wants; you are the dentist and you are the one who makes the decisions. You must show that you are in control and that you are doing what is best for them. They'll thank you for it in the long run. I learnt this at a very early stage of my general practice career, and I never allow myself to be swayed from it.'

'Thank you for the advice, Spencer. What you're saying makes sense.'

'It is the only way, Justin. Patients are always trying to take control of their treatment, asking me to do this or not to do that. They often ask me to rush things through because they want something done for Christmas, or because they are getting married or whatever, but I never give in to their demands. I tell them that if they want me to do the job for them, then it must be done in my way and at my pace. It is one of the few things on which I refuse to be swayed, and I must insist that you follow my instructions on this point. If you try to rush a job through, something always goes wrong, and then what do you do? For example, you have agreed to make a crown for someone at the last minute before their wedding and you find that it doesn't fit properly. What do you do? You haven't time to remake it so you fit it and hope it will be alright. It then fails prematurely a year or two down the line. The patient won't make allowances for the fact that you rushed it through to suit them. They still expect the highest standards, and so you must not do anything which is likely to compromise those standards. You're the boss. Never, never, never, give in to patients' demands.'

'Okay. I'll remember what you said, Spencer, and thanks for the advice. Now, what was it you wanted to talk to me about?'

'As you know, I'm going up to London on Wednesday and won't be back until the weekend. I'm going on a three day dental course, which should be quite interesting and, of course, it is no bad thing to show the Family Health Services Authority and your patients that you are keeping up to date with new developments within the profession. Whilst I'm away, I would be grateful if you would cover for me and see any of my patients who might need emergency treatment.'

'Why yes, of course.'

'There are also one or two patients who tend to come in fairly frequently – more for reassurance than anything else. You may well hear from one of them, if so, I would grateful if you would just see them. There probably won't be much you can actually do for them. As I say, they really come in for reassurance.'

'So do they have dental problems?' I asked, somewhat mystified.

'They do and they don't. There's Mr Archibald, for example, who comes in every day to have his denture eased.'

'Every day!'

'Yes. He has been in every single day since I made the denture for him two years ago. I never actually do anything to it. As you can imagine, if I ground something off it every time he comes to see me there wouldn't be anything left of it by now. He constantly complains of soreness and it's a different place every time. There is never anything to see in his mouth – his gums always look perfectly healthy. Yesterday he was sore at the left side, today it was the right, and tomorrow it will probably be at the front. What I do is look in his mouth and, even though I can't see any soreness, I say "my goodness, Mr Archibald, that looks nasty, but don't worry I'll soon put it right for you". Then I pick up the hand piece and pretend I'm grinding something off the denture. I rinse it under the tap and give it back to him, and he always says it feels much better and goes away happy until next day. If he comes in to see you whilst I'm away, and he probably will, I suggest you do the same. I thought I'd tell you so that you won't waste a lot of time trying to find out what's wrong.'

'Yes, thanks for that, Spencer. Are there any other patients I need to know about?'

'I think you should know about Mrs Duxbury who is likely to drop in on you anytime. She never turns up for appointments that have been arranged for her; she always comes when you aren't expecting her. She came in one day last week, without an appointment. Beryl had difficulty in establishing exactly what her problem was, so I just fitted her in when I had a break between other patients. As Beryl led her into the surgery, Mrs Duxbury said "do you think Mr Padginton will have time to do my hair this morning?" I never did find out whether or not she had a dental problem. She sat in my chair and talked about her sister who has been dead for at least five years, then she said she must go because she wanted to get to the butcher's before he closed for lunch.'

'You certainly seem to have some strange patients, Spencer.'

'I think most practices have a few, but Father seemed to have the knack of attracting them for some reason, and now I'm landed with them. They can be terrible time wasters. It isn't too bad if they are private patients because I bill them for the time they are in the surgery. If they want to sit and talk about their love life instead of letting me get on with their treatment it's fine by me, as long as they pay for the time. The problem comes when they are NHS patients because you don't get paid on a time basis for them. Somehow you have to shut them up and get on with the treatment, which isn't always easy, but if you don't you can be out of pocket.'

'Yes, I have already found that out. Anyway, if I have to see any of your patients I will do what I can for them. I don't mind covering for you whilst you are away, and I hope you have a pleasant time in London.'

'Thanks, Justin. It's good to know that you'll be here to hold the fort whilst I'm away.'

CHAPTER TWENTY-SEVEN

I felt I ought to get to the surgery a bit earlier this morning as I was going to be running the practice in Spencer's absence. He would be well on his way to London and his dental course by now, no doubt drinking coffee and reading *The Times* on the train.

Admittedly, it wasn't an earth shattering achievement for me to be in charge whilst he was away, but somehow the prospect made me feel just that little bit more important, especially as Spencer had made a point of telling me that he had every confidence in my ability to look after things whilst he was away and also said that he felt much easier about going away now that I was on the scene. His holiday was approaching and that would be for two weeks. The next three days would probably give me a foretaste of what to expect when I was left in sole charge. He said that if I hadn't been there it would have been difficult for him to get away for two weeks, as he would have had to try and find a locum to look after the practice and locums are not only difficult to find but are also expensive to employ.

I was just going out of the door of my cottage when the phone rang. I really felt I didn't have time to answer it but if I hadn't I would have spent all morning wondering who had called, so I went back and picked up the handset.

'Hello?'

'Oh hello, Justin, it's Annette here. I was hoping I would catch you before you left for work. I hope you don't mind my phoning you.'

'No, not at all, Annette. What can I do for you?'

'You know I work for the Southern Bank? Well, it's their annual dinner this Saturday and I was wondering if you would consider accompanying me? It is held at the Stonehaven Hotel which, if you don't know it, is a lovely country hotel about five miles from Luccombury. It's a super place and the food is very good. I had lunch there about a month ago and I can thoroughly recommend it. I haven't been to one of the bank's dinners before but I am told they are usually very enjoyable. There will be a champagne reception followed by a five-course meal and there is an after-dinner speaker. As an employee, I automatically receive two tickets. At first I said I wouldn't be going as I didn't have anyone to go with, and then I thought about asking you. I hope you don't mind.'

'Er no, not at all, Annette. Thank you for asking me, but I assume it will be evening dress and I don't have an evening suit.'

'Er...yes, I think it is evening dress, but you could hire one. Please say you will come, Justin.'

'Well, all right. Yes, I will come, and thank you once again for the invitation.'

'Oh, Justin, that's wonderful. Thank you so much. I shall really look forward to it. I'll let you get off to work now and I must do the same, but I will contact you again before Saturday to arrange where and when to meet. Bye, and thank you once again for agreeing to come with me.'

I put down the phone, wondering if I had made the right decision. I had never been particularly keen on wearing evening suits and attending formal dinners at which there would be lots of people; I much preferred an informal setting with one or two close friends. I hardly knew Annette and it was most unlikely that I would know anyone else there. It was nice of her to invite me to accompany her, though perhaps it was in desperation because she couldn't think of anyone else to ask. Anyway I had accepted now, so I was committed.

As soon as I reached the surgery other matters took my mind off the dinner. Beryl told me that two of Spencer's patients had phoned already because they had problems, and she had fitted them into my busy morning schedule. Looking at my appointment book it seemed unlikely that I would be getting a coffee break. Fortunately, Ingrid had also arrived early and with characteristic efficiency had set up everything I needed for my first patient. We were soon under way, and with Ingrid's help I was able to keep more or less on time for most of the morning.

The first of Spencer's emergency patients turned out to be Mr Archibald who, predictably, was complaining of extreme soreness under his denture.

'Thank you for seeing me, Mr Derwent. I couldn't have gone on a moment longer with this. I am in agony. The plate digs right into me on this side every time I close my teeth together, and eating is completely out of the question.'

'Come and sit down and let me have a look, Mr Archibald.

He flopped into my chair and removed his denture without being asked to do so, then he thrust his huge first finger into his mouth in order to indicate the area that was giving trouble. He tried to carry on speaking to me, but the presence of his finger under his tongue made it impossible for me to decipher what he was trying to say.

'Can I have a look, Mr Archibald?' I asked of him, thinking that he would remove his finger in order to let me see, but he didn't. He carried on speaking and this time I was just about able to make out what he said.

'It's down here, Mr Derwent. Can you see it?'

'Will you remove your finger, please?'

'I'm just trying to show you where it hurts.'

'I know, but I can't see into your mouth with your finger there. If you let me examine your gum, I will be able to see where it is sore.'

He removed his finger and I carried out a complete examination. As Spencer had predicted there was not a trace of soreness or ulceration. I couldn't even detect an area of redness on the gum, which would indicate that the denture was rubbing.

'Oh yes, I can see the spot, Mr Archibald. It looks really sore,' I lied, following Spencer's instructions. 'Don't worry, I'll soon solve the problem for you. Give me your denture and I'll ease the flange, then it won't dig into your gum.'

Mr Archibald handed me his plate and I looked at it carefully. 'It's this area here that needs trimming back,' I announced, continuing with the deception. I picked up my slow drill and pretended to grind away some of the plastic. I stopped, examined it closely then pretended to take off a bit more.

'That should do the trick,' I declared rinsing the denture under the tap before handing it back to the patient.

Mr Archibald slipped it back into his mouth. He remained in the chair for some moments as his tongue explored the borders of the denture. It was some time before he spoke.

'That's amazing, Mr Derwent.'

'Really, Mr Archibald? Why do you say that?'

'Well, the denture feels a lot more comfortable, but I would have sworn that you didn't actually grind anything off it.'

'You saw me doing it.'

'I saw you pick up the drill and start it up, but it makes a different noise when it's actually grinding something and usually you can see the dust flying off. I didn't see any dust at all.'

I was about to try and talk my way out of the situation and I began to feel a little uncomfortable at his astute observations. Fortunately it wasn't necessary because he quickly continued.

'Anyway, no matter. It feels much better so I assume you removed the merest whisker. I suppose it's a case of knowing exactly where to take it from; if you get the right spot you don't need to remove very much. When Mr Padginton eases it he grinds loads off and the dust flies everywhere, but probably he isn't as careful as you to make sure he's got the right spot. He probably removes more than is necessary. I am obliged to you, Mr Derwent, for taking the trouble to locate the troublesome area with such accuracy. Thank you very much. Good day.'

'Good day, Mr Archibald. Mr Padginton will be back on Monday, but I shall be happy to help you out if you have any more trouble before then.'

I was puzzled by what Mr Archibald had said. Spencer maintained that he didn't actually grind anything off the denture, but Mr Archibald obviously took careful notice of what went on and said that when Spencer eased the denture there was lots of dust created. It was also true that the drill made a different noise when it was actually grinding something. I decided to go and ask Beryl about it to see if she could offer an explanation.

'I can answer that one for you, Justin,' she said without hesitation. 'Spencer carries a piece of plastic in his pocket and grinds a bit off that instead of Mr Archibald's denture. To begin with, he just used to go through the motions of drilling like you did. Mr Archibald always said that the denture felt more comfortable afterwards, even though Spencer hadn't done anything to it but then one day, for some reason, Mr Archibald said it didn't feel any better and he didn't think Spencer had actually done anything to it on that occasion. Ever since then Spencer has had a piece of plastic with him so that Mr Archibald can be in no doubt that he has done some grinding.'

'The cunning old fox!'

'I suppose when you have been in practice for some time, like Spencer, you learn a few tricks,' laughed Beryl as she returned to her paperwork.

Spencer's second 'emergency' patient was Mrs Tricker, a very round, elderly lady with a face like the harvest moon. She came in to see me just before lunch and she too had a denture problem.

'I am beginning to think that very few people in this part of Dorset have any of their own teeth,' remarked Ingrid, who was amazed at the number of denture patients we had in the practice.

'I suppose it is because there are a lot of old people round here. Many of them move out this way when they retire, and a lot of the local country folk don't bother much with their teeth when they are young and then they have to have them all removed.'

'People in Germany take much better care of their teeth. I don't think there are so many people with dentures.'

'You may well be right, Ingrid, I don't know, but it is certainly true that denture work takes up much of our time here. Anyway, go and fetch Mrs Tricker from the waiting room and let's see what her problem is.'

It took some time for Mrs Tricker's rotund shape to negotiate the stairs and she finally deposited herself into my chair, puffing and blowing. It was immediately obvious from the sunken appearance of her lips and cheeks that she was not wearing her dentures.

'What can I do for you, Mrs Tricker?' I asked.

'It's nice of you to see me, Mr Derwent. Perhaps I should tell you that I have had trouble with my teeth for a long time. They are loose, you see. I haven't much gum, it's all shrunk away. I just can't keep the teeth in. The upper plate drops and the lower moves about all the time and lifts when I talk. Eating is hopeless. Mr Padginton has made me several different plates, but none of them have been any good. Anyway, about two months ago he said to me that he thought he had found a solution to my problem. He sounded quite excited about it, said he had been reading up and had found a way of keeping the teeth in place. He felt sure it would work for me, so he made me this latest set which he fitted for me last week.'

'Really? That's interesting. Loose dentures can be a real problem for some people and I wasn't aware that there is an easy answer. What exactly was Mr Padginton's solution?'

'Springs, Mr Derwent.'

'Springs?'

'Yes, springs.'

Mrs Tricker removed the dentures from her handbag and carefully unpeeled the tissue in which they were wrapped. The first thing I noticed about them was the presence of quite large gold coil springs, one at each side, joining the upper and lower dentures together. The springs were arranged so that they pushed the dentures apart, the idea obviously being that the force of the springs kept the upper denture up and pressed the lower denture down.

'That's ingenious, Mrs Tricker. Come to think of it, I can recall reading somewhere about the use of springs to keep dentures in place, but I thought it was just a bit of a gimmick that was used towards the end of the last century and abandoned because it wasn't very successful.'

'Mr Padginton told me it was a well-tried technique and usually very effective.'

'What do you think? Has it worked for you?'

'I'm not sure. The main problem is that the plates are permanently joined together by the springs, which means that I have to put the top and bottom into my mouth at the same time and my lips just aren't elastic enough. I've split the corners of my mouth trying. Mr Padginton seemed to manage it, but he had a real struggle and it was very painful. I kept the plates in for three days because I didn't think I would be able to get them out. I finally managed it, but now I can't get them back in again.'

'Do they need to be permanently joined together? If you could separate them you could put the dentures in one at a time and then connect up the springs afterwards.'

'Mr Padginton didn't think I would be able to manage to attach the springs if I did it that way. He thought it was better to have the plates permanently joined together. He said that my mouth would stretch eventually and I wouldn't have any difficulty, but it doesn't seem to be getting any easier.'

'How were the dentures when you were wearing them? Did they stay in place?'

'They did, but the springs at the sides felt very big and rubbed against the inside of my cheeks making them sore, and I felt all the time as though my mouth was being forced open. It took a lot of effort to overcome the force of the springs to close my mouth, and after a while my jaw felt very tired. Perhaps the springs are too strong.'

'I have to admit, Mrs Tricker, that I haven't any experience of dentures with springs, so I don't think I can advise you. I don't know if it is possible to obtain different strength springs. You will have to ask Mr Padginton about that. I will try and put the dentures back in for you if you would like me to.'

'I don't think I would, Mr Derwent. It's an awful feeling when you want to take them out because they are uncomfortable but you can't get them out without splitting the corners of your mouth. I think I will wait until Mr Padginton gets back and ask him if he can fit weaker springs. and perhaps think about separating the plates so that I can put them in one at a time.'

'I'm sorry I can't be of more help to you.'

'No matter, Mr Derwent. Thank you for seeing me.'

I was sorry that I was unable to help Mrs Tricker, but dentures with springs were something I had never seen before and I didn't want to do anything which might make matters worse for her. She would have to wait until Spencer got back, though I had a strong suspicion that the idea of fitting springs was one he had come up with in sheer desperation because everything else had failed. It was my guess that this was the first time he had ever used the technique, and his knowledge and experience of it was probably as limited as mine.

The rest of the day passed uneventfully thanks to Ingrid's assistance. I felt we were now becoming an efficient team and I enjoyed dentistry much more as a result. I had never really had this sort of working relationship with a nurse before. When I was a student, I worked with different nurses all the time and I hadn't been with Anna long enough to build up the same rapport. I began to realise just how dependent a dentist becomes on his nurse and that having established this sort partnership it would be a major setback if anything were to bring it to an end.

We were about to clear away after the last patient of the day when Beryl came in looking slightly ruffled.

'Mrs Johnson has just phoned. She has been a patient of the practice for many years and can be a difficult woman. She is very fussy. She broke a front crown on her cereal at breakfast this morning and has waited until now to phone. She wants to see someone about it immediately so I have told her to come straight round. I hope you don't mind, Justin.'

'No I don't mind, but people are a bit inconsiderate, aren't they? She could have phoned earlier.'

I didn't have long to wait for Mrs Johnson. I was looking out of the window and saw her car zoom to a standstill outside. It seemed most unlikely that she had adhered to the speed limit to get here.'

'Thank you so much for seeing me, Mr Derwent. It's very kind of you.'

'That's all right, Mrs Johnson. Come through to my surgery. I understand from Beryl that you have broken a front crown.'

'Yes, that's right, I did it on some breakfast cereal this morning. I wasn't going to bother you with it today but then my husband phoned up this afternoon and said that he wanted me to go with him to meet some business colleagues this evening. I can't possibly go looking like this.'

She lifted her lip to reveal the fact that most of one of her front crowns was missing and she had a very unsightly gap.

'I see what you mean. I will remove what's left of the crown and fit a temporary one. You will need to be very careful with it though, because it will be a plastic one and not very strong, but at least it will restore your appearance.'

'Thank you, Mr Derwent. How soon can you make me a new permanent crown?'

'As you are Mr Padginton's patient you will need to see him to get a new permanent crown. I suggest you make an appointment to see him when he gets back next week.'

'Next week! That's no good. I'm flying off to New Zealand on Saturday. I can't possibly go off with a temporary crown. Can't you fit me a new permanent one before then?'

'I'm sorry, Mrs Johnson, it's out of the question. You are Mr Padginton's patient and it would be unethical for me to do more than is absolutely necessary to get you out of trouble, so all I can do is to fit you with a temporary crown to get you by. In any case, it takes at least a week to get a crown made by the laboratory, so even if Mr Padginton were here we still couldn't make a new crown for you before Saturday.'

'That's rubbish. I'm sure Mr Padginton has made crowns for me in two days previously. I can remember him phoning the technician at the laboratory where the crowns are made and arranging to get the job rushed through.'

'I don't think so, Mrs Johnson. Mr Padginton has a very strict rule that he won't allow himself to deviate from his normal procedure simply to comply with patients' demands.'

'I'm telling you that he has made crowns for me quickly in the past, but as he isn't here anyway, I'm asking you to make the crown for me. I'm a private patient, you know, and I am perfectly willing to pay extra because you are doing the job more quickly.'

'It's not a question of money, Mrs Johnson. Mr Padginton told me only yesterday that I must never submit to pressure from patients and that I must always, *always,* follow practice procedure. I would like to help you, but it isn't my practice and I must comply with Mr Padginton's instructions, even if I don't necessarily agree with them. I know it isn't what you want to hear, but I'm afraid that is the way it is.'

'So you won't help me?'

'I can fit you with a temporary crown, but I cannot arrange for a permanent crown to be made before Saturday.'

'Well don't bother! I shall go somewhere else. I am sure there is a dentist somewhere around here who will make me a crown.'

With that, Mrs Johnson stormed out, slammed the door of her car and left a considerable amount of rubber on the road as she set off with wheels spinning.

'I felt awful about that,' I said to Ingrid, 'but Spencer and I were talking yesterday and he told me that I must never give in to patients' demands. He was quite adamant about it. As he pointed out, if I did try to get the crown made, it is possible that it wouldn't fit properly. For some reason things have a tendency to go wrong when it is important that they don't, and if it doesn't fit you are really in trouble because there is no time to get it remade. Spencer is probably right but Mrs Johnson didn't seem to share his point of view.'

'No, she wasn't at all happy, but I can understand that you have to follow Spencer's instructions,' said Ingrid.

CHAPTER TWENTY-EIGHT

I must admit that Annette looked quite stunning as she came out of her house and walked to my car. Her long kingfisher blue evening dress didn't help her to climb into it as gracefully as perhaps she would have liked, and I tried to alleviate any awkwardness she might be feeling by telling her that small sports cars were quite difficult to get in and out of at the best of times. I held the door open for her as an act of chivalry but stopped short at picking up her feet and guiding them into the foot well.

'I'm so glad you could come with me, Justin. I have been looking forward to this evening all week. I must say, you look very smart in your evening suit.'

'Thank you, Annette. I don't wear one very often and I feel a bit conspicuous in it. It isn't mine – I hired it – but I think it fits quite well. I have to say you look very nice.'

'Why, thank you, Justin. It is a long time since I got dressed up to go out, so I tried to make an effort. I don't think I've been anywhere that called for me to dress up like this since the day I was supposed to get married.'

I could see a look of unhappiness come over her as she spoke, and I thought it wise to try and change the subject as quickly as possible. I didn't want her bursting into tears after spending what must have been a fair amount of time putting on her make-up.

'I think we are quite early. What do you want to do? We could carry on and risk being the first there, or we could go for a little drive somewhere to kill time, or we could stop off and have a drink in a pub on the way.'

'Can we just go for a drive somewhere, Justin? I love your car. I haven't been in a sports car before. I'll bet it's great with the hood down.'

'It's lovely when the weather is good, but it has to be really hot if you are going to drive any distance otherwise there's an icy blast on your head and after a while you feel as if someone has chopped the top of your head off.'

Annette laughed at the thought and I was relieved that I appeared to have snapped her out of her moment of sadness.

'I'd ask you to put the hood down now but I can't risk having my hair blown about. Perhaps you'll put it down when we drive home tonight? It will be fun coming home in the dark with the wind rushing through our hair. It will also help to clear our heads if we have had a bit too much to drink.'

'I can assure you that as I shall be driving you home, I shall be very careful not to have too much to drink.'

'It's very kind of you to offer to drive, though it's a shame that you won't be able to drink very much. We could have got a taxi.'

'I don't mind driving. I don't really drink very much anyway, and I certainly don't like having too much. It's not that long ago we had a party at the practice because a nurse was leaving and my boss got me well and truly drunk. I felt bad for about two days and vowed that I would never do it again.'

'Well, I hope the fact that you can't drink won't spoil your enjoyment of the evening.'

'No, it won't, Annette.'

It was a warm and pleasant evening and we took a leisurely drive through the rolling hills of the Dorset countryside. The low sun was casting long and picturesque shadows and I regretted leaving my camera at home. As well as the possibility of interesting landscapes, I thought that some portraits of Annette in her evening dress in a country setting could have been most attractive. I personally would have been very happy to drive down to the coast and call in at a country pub for some food instead of going to a formal dinner where I would be surrounded by lots of people I didn't know. Obviously that was out of the question as plans for the evening had been made. I didn't want Annette to know that I had very mixed feelings about going to the bankers' dinner so I didn't say anything to her.

'Well, here we are, Annette,' I said to her as we drew up in the Stonehaven Hotel car park. 'I'll open the door and help you out of the car.'

'It's a very long time since a gentleman assisted me in and out of his car, Justin. I feel very honoured.'

'I'm not sure I deserve the "gentleman" title.'

'Well you are behaving like a gentleman, so you deserve to be referred to as one.'

We entered the hotel foyer and were directed to the suite where the dinner was being held. There were already quite a number of people there chatting in groups and most of them were clutching glasses of champagne. What struck me immediately, however, causing me some concern, was the fact that all the men were wearing lounge suits. None of them was wearing a formal evening suit. Many of the women were in long dresses, so Annette was quite appropriately dressed, but I felt sure that I would stick out like a sore thumb and I began to feel very self-conscious.

'You said it was evening dress,' I said to Annette.

'I thought it was. I am terribly sorry if I got it wrong, Justin, but you look so handsome dressed like that. I am sure it doesn't really matter. It is better to be overdressed than underdressed at something like this.'

'I told you I feel conspicuous in evening dress. I certainly shall if I am the only one wearing it.'

Annette was clearly upset that her mistake had made me feel uncomfortable. She snuggled up close to me and squeezed my hand.

'I really appreciate you coming with me this evening, Justin. I wouldn't have come without you and you look fabulous in your evening suit. I am very proud to have you with me and you must not feel the slightest bit awkward.'

I began to feel a bit guilty that I was making such a fuss about it. Annette was probably right in that nobody really took any notice.

'I'm sorry, Annette, you're right. It doesn't matter. I won't think any more about it. Now, can I get you a drink?'

'Thank you. I would love some champagne but I must warn you it goes to my head very quickly.'

I didn't need to search for a drink, because no sooner had I mentioned it than a waiter came over with a tray. We both took a glass.

'There's my boss, Mr Fitzpatrick, over there, Justin. Come on I'll introduce you to him.'

Mr Fitzpatrick was a tall, thin man with a small moustache that looked almost as if it had been painted on to his upper lip. He had a hooked nose and a pointed chin, and his slightly greying hair was parted just left of centre. As soon as he saw Annette his face lit up and he turned away from the group he was with to welcome her.

'Annette, my dear you look absolutely wonderful. Come here and give me a kiss. I am so glad you were able to come after all.'

Annette walked up to him and Mr Fitzpatrick put his arms around her and kissed her on the cheek. His enthusiasm for the embrace clearly outweighed Annette's, but she didn't offend him.

'I want you to meet Justin,' she announced.

'I'm very pleased to meet you, Justin.' We shook hands and soon the rest of Mr Fitzpatrick's group joined us.

'This is Mr Taylor,' Annette said, introducing me to the shortest male member of the group. 'He and I work together.'

He held out his hand to me, 'Hello, Justin, call me Roger.' Turning to Annette he asked, 'is Justin your boyfriend?'

Annette hesitated before replying. 'Er yes, yes he is.'

'You lucky fellow, Justin. I can tell you there are quite a few members of the bank who have had their eyes on Annette ever since she came to work with us, but none of us has succeeded in cracking her shell so far. You must be very special.'

'He is,' confirmed Annette, clutching my arm as if we had been in a close relationship for a very long time.

I refrained from saying that until a few moments ago I hadn't been aware that Annette considered me to be her boyfriend and that I had never looked upon her as my girlfriend. I decided that this was not the time nor the place to mention it and I just let it go.

'Are you connected with banking, Justin?' enquired Mr Fitzpatrick politely.

'No he's a dental surgeon,' Annette blurted out proudly before I had time to reply. She didn't give me the chance to follow

Spencer's advice about not declaring to strangers the nature of one's profession.

'Good grief,' Roger exclaimed. 'You look quite a gentle sort of chap. I can't believe that you would want to inflict pain on people. It just goes to show that appearances can be deceptive.'

'He is gentle,' Annette interjected defensively.

'I don't see how he can be,' said Roger. 'All dentists are sadists – they must be to do the job in the first place.'

'That's rubbish,' Annette retorted. 'You think what it would be like if there weren't any dentists and we all had rotten teeth and had to suffer terrible toothache.'

'Tell me, Justin,' Mr Fitzpatrick intervened, looking serious. 'Why is that whenever I go for treatment the dentist fills my mouth with all sorts of gadgets and instruments and then expects me to answer a load of questions?'

I couldn't believe that Spencer's analysis could be so accurate. I didn't answer Mr Fitzpatrick's question straight away. I just waited to see if anyone moved on to complete phase three. Roger prevented me from being disappointed.

'I can remember when I had to have a wisdom tooth removed. The roots were hooked like claws and it took the best part of an hour and a half to get it out. Sweat was pouring from the dentist, even though he was a huge rugby player. God knows how many stitches he had to put in and I swelled up like a balloon. I couldn't open my mouth for a week afterwards and I had to live on liquids. It was a hell of an experience. I would never go through it again. I would rather live with permanent toothache.'

'You say that now, but if you had severe toothache you would be glad to see a dentist,' continued Annette, steadfast in defending me. 'I think it must be a very demanding job and I admire everyone in that sort of profession – dentists, doctors and nurses.'

'Well you would say that, he's your boyfriend,' Roger quipped. Perhaps I was reading too much into the situation but I got the impression that Roger quite fancied Annette and had thought that she was unattached. My presence had come as a disappointment to him, especially as Annette had introduced me as her boyfriend.

The room slowly filled and, as I feared, I was the only man in an evening suit. No-one actually said anything but I felt that many people looked at me and wondered why I was so overdressed. Waiters circulated the room with trays of champagne, and empty glasses were exchanged for full ones. I was mindful of the fact that I would be driving home, and strictly limited my intake. I had no idea who else in our group was driving, but from where I was standing it seemed that none of them felt constrained to go easy on the alcohol. Annette was certainly draining her glass at an alarming rate.

Eventually we were called in to dinner and we filtered through to the spacious dining room, which was laid out with about twenty round tables each dressed with a spotless white table cloth and adorned with a colourful vase of flowers. The seating had been arranged by departments which meant that Annette and I, Mr Fitzpatrick and his wife, and Roger Taylor were all on the same table. We were joined by a small middle-aged lady called Jean, who worked with Annette, and her husband, Raymond. Jean was obviously shortsighted and wore very thick spectacles which shrunk her eyes to the size of tiny beads, whilst her husband must have suffered from the opposite ophthalmic defect and had glasses which greatly magnified his eyes. The eighth and final member of the party was a timid little man called Hugh whose face was so pale he looked as if he had never been out in the sun in his life. His dark brown hair was plastered down with hair cream and he had a very distracting nervous twitch at the corner of his mouth when he was speaking.

Because there was a sex imbalance at our table, it was not possible for every person to be flanked by two members of the opposite sex and I found myself seated between Jean and Hugh. Annette was on the opposite side of the table between Roger and Raymond.

The food turned out to be first class and glasses of champagne were replaced with glasses of excellent wine. Jean was very pleasant and she and I engaged in conversation about all sorts of subjects, but as soon as we discovered that we were both interested in photography that became our main topic for discussion. Much as I enjoyed talking to Jean, I was aware that Hugh on my left was being left out of things because Mr Fitzpatrick, who was sitting on the other side of him, spent most of the time talking to Raymond. I tried to divide my attention and spent much of the main course talking to Hugh, but in doing so, I discovered one of the other features about being a dentist of which one had to be wary – something that Spencer had not warned me about.

Hugh was present when Annette announced that I was a dentist and he couldn't wait to talk to me about his very profound and deep-seated fear of dentistry – a fear that had prevented him from visiting a dentist for the past eighteen years. He was worried that he might need a lot of treatment. In fact, he was well-aware that he had a number of holes in his teeth, but fear prevented him from arranging an appointment with a dentist.

He had had a few glasses of champagne and was feeling more relaxed. He discovered that, in spite of being a dentist, I appeared to be fairly human and approachable, and this made him feel able to pour out his dental troubles and phobias to me. He could also feel sure that I was not going to ask him to open his mouth there and then. The more we talked the more his confidence grew, helped by the steadily increasing degree of alcohol-induced tranquilization.

Finally he made a surprising statement.

'Justin, I honestly think I would be able to overcome my long-standing fear of dentists sufficiently to come and see you professionally. Talking to you has made me feel confident that you would be kind and understanding and that you would be able to coax me through the necessary treatment. Would you be prepared to see me?'

For a moment I didn't quite know what to say. I was a little flattered that I had succeeded in gaining his confidence, but then I realised that he had consumed quite a lot of champagne and wine and that he might feel very different in the cold light of day when he had sobered up.

'Why, er yes, of course I would be prepared to see you. I suggest you phone the surgery on Monday and arrange an appointment.'

'I don't think I would have the nerve to do that. Can't you give me a day and a time now? Then I would have to come. I never break appointments.'

'It is difficult without my diary.'

'Please, Justin, I will come whenever you say, but if we don't fix up a time now, I know that I won't be brave enough to phone up to arrange it.'

I felt sorry for him and wanted to help so I replied, 'you could come at five o'clock on Monday and I will see you after my last patient. How would that suit you?'

'I had hoped that it could be earlier in the day, then I wouldn't have so long to think about it, but I realise that without your diary it is difficult. All right then, I'll come at five o'clock. I don't think the bank is going to get much work out of me on Monday. I shall be too nervous thinking about coming to see you.'

'Do you know where the practice is?'

'Yes. I have been there several times over the past few years to make an appointment, but on each occasion my courage failed me at the last moment and I couldn't cross the threshold. But now that I have met you and talked to you I don't feel quite so bad about it. I will definitely come on Monday.'

I didn't get to speak to Hugh much after that. I spent some more time talking to Jean, and then it was time for the after-dinner speaker who was someone high up in the banking world and who seemed well-known to everyone except me. His talk was quite entertaining and at times amusing, but it was clearly aimed at members of the banking profession and much of what he said went over the top of my head.

Each time I turned towards Annette she seemed to be looking in my direction and I couldn't help noticing that Roger always seemed to be looking in Annette's direction. He had moved his chair round, ostensibly in order to get a better view of the speaker, but in doing so had moved it closer to Annette. He kept on whispering comments into her ear, some of which made her laugh. There was no doubt in my mind that he was very interested in her but I got the impression from Annette's body language that his feelings were not reciprocated.

Soon after the speaker sat down, Jean and Raymond announced that they ought to leave because they were worried about their dog, who had undergone an operation the previous day and had not yet fully recovered. Raymond's departure had left Annette completely at the mercy of Roger who seemed to be moving forever closer to her, but she stood up somewhat unsteadily and, holding on to the table for support, came round to sit in Jean's seat, next to me.

'I'm so sorry I couldn't sit next to you, Justin. We've hardly spoken to each other all evening,' Annette said, her speech slightly slurred.

'Yes it was a shame, Annette. Did you enjoy the meal?'

'I thought the meal and the wine were good. I'm not so sure about the after-dinner speech though, and I definitely could have done without Roger's attention. Do you know he had the nerve to suggest taking me home?'

'I can tell he likes you.'

'But what a cheek when I had told him you were my boyfriend.'

'Am I?'

'You are a boy, or a young man, and you are my friend, so that makes you my boyfriend doesn't it?'

'I suppose it does,' I replied, not wishing to challenge the logic of Annette's statement, particularly in view of the fact that there was definitely an alcoholic haze clouding her ability to think clearly.

'Let's go home, Justin.'

She clung on to my arm as she rose from her chair. It was partly to steady herself, but there was no doubt she was snuggling up close to me at the same time. I had often heard it said that when you have had too much to drink, as Annette obviously had, as soon as the fresh air hits you, you pass out. I sincerely hoped that Annette would not do so.

In fact, the fresh air seemed to have the reverse effect and by the time we had crossed the car park to my car she seemed less drunk.

'Will you put the hood down please, Justin?'

'I will if you want me to, but it might be a bit cold. You must tell me if it is too draughty for you.'

'I'm sure it won't be. It will be lovely to feel the wind rushing past. I think it is just what I need. I must admit that I overdid the champagne when we first got there.'

'Well, as long as you enjoyed it, that's all that matters.'

'Did you enjoy the evening, Justin? I am sorry that you got landed with Hugh.'

'He was okay. He is coming to see me professionally on Monday. Apparently he hasn't seen a dentist for many years. He told me he is terrified, but feels that he will be able to summon up the courage to see me. I expect it was the drink talking. He will probably feel very different about it when he wakes up tomorrow morning.'

'It was probably because he saw that you are a very kind and caring person like I do. I'll bet you're a wonderful dentist.'

'I don't know about that, Annette.'

'I'm sure you are.'

Annette fell silent for some minutes but there was a look of serenity on her face and she seemed to be enjoying the feel of the wind blowing her hair about. She didn't speak again until I drew up outside her house.

'Oh Justin, we're home already. I was enjoying the ride.'

She looked straight into my eyes and placed her hand on mine. 'Would you like to come and spend the night with me, Justin?'

I wasn't ready for that and I'm not sure whether I was surprised or downright scared.

'It's a lovely thought, Annette,' I responded after a pause, 'but I'm a bit worried that the wine has something to do with the way you are feeling and we might both regret it in the morning. Let me help you out of the car and see you to your door.'

I opened the car door for her and put my arm round her to lift her out of the low seat. As soon as her feet were safely on the ground she turned her face towards mine and planted a soft kiss squarely on my lips.

'Thank you so much for coming with me this evening, Justin, I'm just sorry that we didn't get the opportunity to spend more time alone together.'

'Thank you for inviting me. I enjoyed it, even if I was the only man wearing an evening suit.'

'I'm so sorry about that. Can you ever forgive me?' she replied, laughing.

'I think I can. I am sure much worse things have happened to me in life.'

I walked with her to her door and she fumbled in her handbag for her key. She had some difficulty locating the keyhole so I took the key from her and guided it into the lock. I opened the door and stood back to let her enter the house, an action which must have indicated to her that I didn't intend going in with her.

'Are you sure you won't come in?' she sighed wistfully.

I just nodded and said, 'I had better go.'

I turned and waved to her as I got into my car and she blew a kiss to me.

CHAPTER TWENTY-NINE

It was almost lunchtime the next day when the phone rang.

'Hi Justin. It's me, Annette.'

'Hello Annette. How is your head this morning?'

'Not too good but I've taken some paracetamol and I'm feeling a bit better now. I wanted to say how much I enjoyed being with you last night, and to thank you for coming with me. I don't go out very much these days. In fact, I haven't felt like going out for some time. Last night was the first time in ages, and it was lovely, thanks to you.'

'I am very glad you enjoyed it. It was interesting to meet people from the banking world. It makes a change from being with other dentists all the time. They seem very nice people.'

'I think Jean is nice and Mr Fitzpatrick is all right. Roger can be a bit of pain in the neck.'

'He is obviously attracted to you.'

'Well, I'm not attracted to him, but he doesn't seem to get the message. He has tried it on once or twice at work and when I saw that I had been put next to him on the table I couldn't believe it. I wouldn't be surprised if he arranged that himself.'

'Perhaps he did.'

'I do hope, Justin, that I didn't upset or offend you in any way last night. I realise I had a bit too much to drink and said things that perhaps I shouldn't have. I would hate to think that I did or said anything to make you have a poor opinion of me.'

'No, of course not, Annette. I was very flattered by what you said and I hope that I didn't offend you. What you said came as a bit of a bolt out of the blue, that's all.'

'I said things that I probably wouldn't have said if I hadn't had so much to drink, but I knew what I was saying and I meant it. I have never asked anyone to stay the night with me before but somehow it just felt right with you. I feel that we are getting on so well together and even though we haven't known each other very long there seems to be something special between us.'

'Please don't think that I didn't want to. It's just that I wasn't expecting it, and I was a bit worried that we might be rushing into something we weren't ready for.'

'I can understand that, but it felt right to me. I do hope that we can go out together again. Can we, Justin?'

I hesitated. It wasn't that I didn't want to see Annette. I liked her, she was attractive and intelligent, but I felt she was trying to move things on between us far too quickly.

'Why yes, of course,' I responded somewhat feebly. 'Will you be going to the Bankks Club tomorrow?' Then I remembered that I wouldn't be going as I was attending a dental lecture at Dorchester Hospital. 'I'm sorry Annette, I've just remembered that I can't go tomorrow as I have to go to a lecture, but I will be there next week.'

I thought that a delay of a week might be a good thing because it would give both of us time to reflect upon the way our relationship might be heading. I don't think Annette felt the same way.

'Won't I see you before then?'

I didn't want her to feel that I was giving her the brush –off, but at the same time I felt that I had to slow things down a bit.

'I have a busy week ahead, I'm afraid,' I replied somewhat unconvincingly, then not wishing to hurt her feelings I added, 'I promise I will phone you later in the week if I can get ahead on some of the things I must do.'

'I will wait and hope. I would so like to see you again soon. Promise me you will phone if you possibly can.'

'I promise.'

'Goodbye then, Justin. Take care.'

'Goodbye Annette, and you take care as well.'

The telephone call confirmed to me that Annette was hoping that we might be able to establish some sort of relationship, something more than just friendship, and I wasn't at all sure how I felt about it. It seemed to me that for her it would be very much on the rebound following the breakdown of her engagement. I was also aware that she was extremely vulnerable at this time, and if I upset her emotionally she might not be able to cope.

I was finding my way in general practice and in a new part of the country and I wanted time to settle in and to establish a circle of friends, rather than tie myself down to one person in particular. At present the relationship hadn't really got off the ground, and I wondered if it might be best to call a halt to it here and now. On the other hand, I didn't feel that I could be that blunt with her. I liked her company, she was lonely and also needed friends, so provided we could remain just friends and nothing more, it would be good for both of us.

I thought about it hard and long. I really didn't want to upset Annette, but at the same time I didn't want her to believe that I was ready for anything more than friendship. If I could keep in touch with her but avoid getting into a one-to-one situation, maybe I could keep things under control. I wasn't at all sure. I hadn't really had a deep romantic attachment to anyone so far in my life. I had little or no experience of emotional relationships and I didn't really know what to do for the best.

I finally decided that I would try to carry on as normally as possible. I would not make any major pronouncements to Annette – there was no need to do so. I would be happy to meet her at the Bankks Club meetings, play tennis with her, and go for a drink, but I would avoid leading her to believe that our relationship was anything more than friendship. Would it work? I had no idea. I hadn't enough experience of women to be able to predict how things would turn out. Only time would tell.

CHAPTER THIRTY

Spencer was back. I knew that because I could hear him rushing around in his surgery as I went past his door. I wanted to see how he got on in London and no doubt he would have a lot to tell me about it but I was in a hurry. I was late and I had a busy morning ahead of me. I would talk to him later.

Ingrid was already in my surgery and had set out my instruments for my first patient with her usual efficiency, but as soon as I saw her I could see that she had a problem. She had a piece of tissue in her hand and was looking at herself in a hand mirror. Her left eye was very red and watering copiously.

'Justin,' she called out, 'will you have a look in my eye? A piece of grit flew into it on my way into work this morning. It's very painful.'

'Yes, of course, Ingrid. Let me see.'

I moved her to a position by the window and looked closely into her eye. I could immediately see a large foreign object and rolled a piece of tissue into a point so that I could gently wipe away the offending piece of grit. My face was very close to hers and when Spencer walked into my surgery a moment later he must have thought I was kissing her.

'Justin, what the hell are you up to?' he cried.

I knew immediately what he was thinking. He had convinced himself that I wouldn't be able to keep my hands off Ingrid and now he was sure he had caught us 'in the act'. I smiled to myself and was in no hurry to explain the truth to him. I decided I would let him go on thinking I was up to no good as long as possible. I kept my back to him pretending I hadn't noticed his presence and I said, 'I hope you feel better now, Ingrid.'

'Much better now thank you, Justin,' she replied.

'What the devil is going on here?' Spencer demanded to know.

I turned to face him. 'Oh, hello Spencer. I didn't hear you come in.'

'That's obvious,' he retorted.

Ingrid explained that a piece of grit had blown into her eye and that I had removed it for her. Spencer just grunted as if to say whilst that may be true he couldn't help thinking I had taken advantage of the situation to get closer to Ingrid than I would normally be able to do.

'How was London?' I enquired.

'Great. Absolutely inspirational,' he enthused. 'It is amazing how much one learns at these academic gatherings. You should go to more of them, Justin. You can't afford to rest on your laurels thinking you know it all just because you are qualified. Personally, I can't get enough postgraduate education. I can't wait for the next lecture. It is the only way to keep up to speed in an ever-changing profession. It is so important, in fact we owe it to our patients to give them the benefit of the very latest and most up-to-date treatment, and education is the only way to achieve this. It isn't always convenient for us to give up our spare time to attend these meetings but it must be a priority, otherwise we are not worthy to be called dental surgeons. I know you would prefer to go to the pub or take a girl out, but that must take second place if you are to be a true professional.'

'As a matter of fact, Spencer, I am going to a lecture at Dorchester Hospital this evening. From what you have just said, you would probably like to come with me.'

Spencer started to back-pedal. 'Well, I would have done, but unfortunately I already have something else on this evening.'

'Something that must take priority even over postgraduate education?'

'Er, yes, on this occasion, I'm afraid it must. Anyway I've got something to show you when you get a minute – something very exciting which I think is going to open up a whole new field for us at this practice. I don't know why I didn't think of it before. I got the idea from one of the other dentists on the course. You see, the beauty of these meetings is that not only do you learn from the lectures, but you also learn from your fellow colleagues. As soon as you have a spare ten minutes, pop into my surgery and I will tell you about it.'

I was intrigued to learn about Spencer's new venture but I was so busy during the morning that it was lunchtime before I had a chance to go into his surgery. As soon as our last patient had left, I suggested to Ingrid that we go and catch Spencer before he left for lunch and find out what he was so excited about. As soon as I opened his surgery door I noticed a piece of equipment that I hadn't seen before. It was cream in colour and freestanding with a series of tubes and pipes and gas cylinders. I recognised it immediately as a general anaesthetic machine, though it was somewhat more old-fashioned than the machines they had at the dental hospital.

'Good grief, Spencer. Where did you get that from?'

'My father bought it years ago. It has been up in the loft, but it seems to be in good condition. I have cleaned it up and I am sure it is practically as good as new. There is even gas in the cylinders. Have you used one like this before?'

'The ones we had at the dental hospital were the same make but a bit more modern. This one is a MK II, whilst the ones at the hospital were MK Vs.'

'They are virtually the same,' Spencer reassured me. 'They made some minor modifications, that's all.'

'I hope you aren't thinking that I shall be giving general anaesthetics?' I said anxiously.

'You did them at the hospital, didn't you?'

'Yes. We had to do one gas session every week during our last two years, but everyone, including me, hated it. We had a consultant in charge of us and he was sweetness itself to everyone until the patient was asleep, then he would let rip. He used to swear and curse at us and make us feel complete idiots. By the end of the session you felt totally demoralised. But that's not why I wouldn't want to give an anaesthetic; it's because frankly I think it is downright dangerous. I am amazed that we didn't kill anyone. Giving general anaesthesia in the dental chair is a very specialised field, and one that requires a great deal of skill and experience. I wouldn't do it for all the tea in China. What about you? Surely you don't feel competent to do it, do you?'

'I don't think it is anything like as difficult as you are making out. I would be perfectly happy to give a whiff of gas if necessary. I haven't done it for a good few years, but there really isn't much to it. My father used to give the gas and extract the teeth himself without any assistance.'

I was horrified at what he was saying. 'Oh come on, Spencer, you know that there have been a few cases where patients have died. I am not prepared to risk that by taking part in a procedure that I don't feel adequately qualified to undertake.'

'I am amazed that you don't feel capable of doing it.' continued Spencer pompously. 'I can only conclude that your training was sadly lacking. Anyway, as it turns out, neither of us will have to give the gas because we are lucky enough to have an expert dental anaesthetist right here in Luccombury – Dr Balfour MacKean. Apparently he used to gas for quite a few dental practices all round the area. He hasn't done it for some years because there hasn't been any demand, but it's like riding a bike; once you can do it you never forget. Anyway I phoned him up last night and he has agreed to do a gas session for us if we get the patients together.'

'Is there any demand for it now, here in Luccombury?' I asked doubtfully.

'I am sure there is, Justin. How many times do you get a patient ask if they can just be put out so that they don't know anything about their treatment? There are lots of people out there too nervous to come to see us because they think they are going to get hurt. If they know we will put them to sleep, they will be happy.'

' Giving a patient a whiff of gas to take a tooth out is one thing but carrying out lengthy treatment – fillings, etcetera, under general anaesthetic is something else. Surely you aren't contemplating doing that, are you?' I was appalled at the prospect, which to my mind was a highly dangerous procedure that carried a very substantial risk of the patient coming to harm.

'No, Justin, of course not. Well, not at the moment, anyway. The treatment will be limited to extractions, but there are still lots of people who know they need to have a tooth extracted but are terrified of having it done whilst they are awake. I can see this as a real money-spinner. It will all be done privately, except, of course, for children who I am happy to see under the National Health, and we can charge the adults a good fee. In addition, it gives our practice an extra string to its bow, so to speak. It will be a worthwhile addition to the wide range of treatments we already provide, and I am sure that patients will appreciate it. Once word gets around that we can offer this service, I expect it will snowball because there aren't many practices in this area doing it. In fact, I can't think of any. As you know, if a patient needs a general anaesthetic, the only way at present is to refer them to the hospital and they have to wait ages before they get an appointment. Who knows, it may well be that other practices will refer patients to us.'

I found it difficult to share Spencer's optimism. As far as I was concerned, my experience of general anaesthesia at the dental hospital had been enough to put me off for life. It conjured up memories of multiple extractions on patients with badly neglected mouths – a very bloody and unpleasant experience – and children being sick.

However, Spencer's enthusiasm was boundless. 'As I said,' he continued, 'I got the idea from a colleague. He started doing G.A.s about five years ago, and now he has a whole morning session every week. He gets referrals from other practices and has built up a good reputation for the service. I am hoping that we will be able to do the same here. I see this as a niche just waiting to be filled and we have everything needed to fill it. So what I want you to do, Justin, is to spread the word among your patients that we are about to introduce this service at the practice. I have fixed the date of the first session for next Monday morning. Balfour is coming here about nine thirty, and we hope to get the first patient in the chair at ten o'clock, so try to book in as many patients as you can for this session.'

'A week doesn't give us much time to fill the session. Frankly I can't think of any of my patients who would be interested in coming for a general anaesthetic, but I will ask.'

'Justin, why are you being so negative about this? I think it will work extremely well. I already have two patients booked in. One is a middle-aged man who has been putting off having a lower molar extracted for about four years because he once had a bad experience when an injection didn't work properly. He keeps on having to take antibiotics and suffers bouts of severe pain every two or three months. He can't wait to come. The other is a little girl who has severe crowding and needs four teeth out for orthodontic purposes. In this sort of situation, I never think it is fair to a child to take out all four teeth in one go because you have to give them so many injections, but this way she won't know anything about it. It is so much kinder.'

I thought about the time I had 'gas' to have a tooth extracted when I was about eight years old. The memory of it still brings me out in a cold sweat and I considered it to be one of the most horrific experiences of my life. I said to Spencer, 'have you ever had gas at the dentist?'

'No. When I had to have teeth out, my father insisted on doing it by injection, but it was very unpleasant. Children don't like having teeth out by injection.'

'Children don't like having teeth out at all, but I can tell you from personal experience that having gas is not just unpleasant – it is absolutely dreadful.'

'You have had a tooth extracted under general anaesthetic, have you?'

'Yes when I was about eight. It was the most awful experience imaginable. I can still smell the rubber mask as it was placed over my face. In fact, for years afterwards just the smell of a rubber object could make me physically sick. And when you come round you feel unbelievably bad. It is the sort of experience to put someone off going to the dentist for life.'

'Oh come on, Justin, you are exaggerating. It couldn't have put you off dentistry that much, or you wouldn't have become a dentist yourself.'

'I probably became a dentist to save people from that sort of horrific experience. I vowed that I would never make a patient of mine suffer what I suffered.'

'What about you, Ingrid. Have you ever had gas?'

'No and I don't think any of my friends have either. Perhaps the dentists in Germany don't use gas. I don't really know, but it sounds quite a good idea that patients just go to sleep and then wake up when the treatment is all over, especially for those patients who are nervous.'

'Exactly,' cried Spencer, 'what a sensible girl she is, Justin. I really can't understand why you are so opposed to this.'

'Unless you have experienced it for yourself, you cannot imagine just how horrible it is. However, it appears that your mind is made up. I will inform my patients that we are now going to be providing this service, and if any of them decide they want to avail themselves of it then fine.'

'Well, I hope you try to promote it. If we are to get Balfour MacKean here on a regular basis, we will need to find the patients to fill the sessions.'

With that, Spencer took off his operating coat and hung it up on the door. I took this as an indication that the conversation had come to an end and that he was going to lunch.

'I am very concerned about this,' I said to Ingrid after he had left.

'Why do you say that? Surely Spencer knows what he is doing, and he won't be giving the general anaesthetic himself. Dr MacKean will be doing that.'

'Exactly. I went to Dr MacKean's for an insurance medical and frankly I wasn't all that impressed with what I saw. You think Spencer's surgery is out of date? You should see Dr MacKean's. I think he might also be a bit behind the times with his methods, and Spencer said he hadn't done any dental anaesthetics for some years. Put Spencer and Dr MacKean together and it could be a recipe for disaster.'

'I do hope not,' said Ingrid seriously.

'So do I, but Spencer seems determined to go ahead. Personally, I shall have as little to do with it as possible.'

Every time I went past Spencer's surgery door I could hear him extolling the virtues of general anaesthesia to his patients, desperately trying to drum up business for the first 'gas' session on Monday morning. My approach was somewhat different. My policy was to say absolutely nothing about it to anyone, in spite of Spencer's request for me to try to 'sell' it to patients, but by pure coincidence one young man raised the subject with me. During the course of his treatment he said that he would much prefer to be unconscious and thought it would be wonderful to wake up and find that it was all over. I was prepared to ignore the comment, but Ingrid stepped in.

'You should tell Mr Strange that we are going to be doing treatment under general anaesthetic from next Monday.' She looked at me and smiled mischievously as she spoke.

'Is that right, Mr Derwent? If so, perhaps we ought to postpone my treatment today and arrange for me to be put out. I'd much prefer it.'

'We will only be carrying out extractions. We won't be able to do fillings or other treatment under general anaesthetic.'

'Why not? I said I wanted to be put out but I don't want to wake up with no teeth.'

'You can only keep someone anaesthetised safely for a very short time in the dental chair. It wouldn't be long enough to do fillings. It becomes dangerous if you try to maintain the anaesthesia for longer than a few minutes.'

'Why is that?'

'It is all to do with blocking off the throat to make sure that nothing gets into the lungs. We can only achieve that safely for a very short time. If we tried to do fillings, there would be too great a risk of bits of filling material going down the throat.'

'How do they manage it in hospitals? They do all sorts of things there.'

'A qualified anaesthetist can block off the throat completely to make sure that nothing goes down, but before you can do that you have to pass a tube into the wind-pipe.'

'Well, can't you do that?'

'No, not really. Dentists aren't trained to do that.'

'It doesn't sound as though I am going to be able to get the treatment I need then, does it?'

'I'm afraid not, Mr Strange.'

'But you may know someone who wants to be put to sleep to have a tooth out,' Ingrid added, knowing full well that I was unlikely to mention it.

'I can't think of anyone off hand, but I'll bear it in mind,' said Mr Strange.

That was the only occasion during the week that the topic of general anaesthesia was brought up in my surgery. At the end of the week I was eager to find out whether Spencer had managed to add to the list for the Monday session.

'Unfortunately, no,' was his answer. 'But it is early days yet and I think that most people would want a bit more notice. Monday is probably too soon because it is less than a week away. However, I have every confidence that we will soon have them flocking in for the service. I suggest that we fix up a date for the next session for about a month's time and that will give us lots of time to fill it.'

'Is it worth getting Balfour MacKean here just for two patients? Presumably you are going to have to pay him a fee for the session, irrespective of the number of patients? Two patients, one of them a child on National Health, isn't even going to cover his fee, is it?'

'Well, actually, it's just one patient now.' Spencer looked somewhat crest-fallen. 'The little girl's parents have heard from somewhere that general anaesthetic carries a risk, and they have decided they would rather not take that risk. They want their daughter's teeth extracted by injection instead.'

'Well, surely it isn't worth it then for just one patient. Why don't you cancel Monday altogether and aim at starting in a month's time?'

'It isn't all about money, Justin. This is just the beginning of a new venture, and we must be patient. The fact that there will only be one patient doesn't matter at all. It will give us a chance to get to know Balfour and how he works and there will be a lot to discuss so that we can organise ourselves in the future. I'm looking forward to it and you should be too.'

The truth was that I wasn't looking forward to it. Maybe I had been put off the idea of general anaesthesia by my own experience at the age of eight and the weekly sessions at the dental hospital when I was a student. Whatever the reason, I intended to play as little part as possible in Spencer's new venture.

The more I thought about it the more concerned I became. It was true that there had been one or two tragic accidents caused by dentists giving general anaesthetics in their surgeries, and the authorities were becoming a bit twitchy about it. It was certainly no longer acceptable for a dentist to give the anaesthetic and extract the teeth himself; there had to be another qualified person present. As Balfour – a qualified medical practitioner was going to be giving the anaesthetic, then surely everything would be fine.

It was just that I was not totally convinced that Balfour and Spencer together amounted to a competent team. Although I intended to remain in the sidelines as far as possible, I couldn't help worrying about it and the prospect of the first general anaesthetic session next Monday occupied my thoughts for most of the time.

In addition to this, my other concern was that Annette telephoned me every evening that week and she began to make me feel a bit claustrophobic. It was true that I had half-promised to phone her, but she wasn't prepared to wait for me to do that and was trying to speed things along. Unfortunately, the more she pestered me, the less inclined I felt to go out with her. I was sure that she was looking for a serious relationship, but as it was going to be very much 'on the rebound', I felt most uncomfortable about it. Perhaps it was conceited of me to think it, but she had given all the signs of wanting to become deeply involved. First of all, I thought that we didn't yet know each other well enough for that, and if we did form a relationship and that relationship were to fail, it might hurt her very badly and she might not be strong enough to take it. I didn't want to be the one to hurt her.

I found talking to her on the phone very difficult. I was fond of her and very much wanted to remain friendly, and I hoped that maybe we could go out together occasionally, perhaps with other people. I had to try to encourage our friendship, but at the same time avoid leading her to believe there was any more in it than that without upsetting her. It was like walking a tightrope and I wasn't at all sure I could retain my balance. I somehow managed to convince her that I had a busy week and that I had genuine reasons for not phoning her, even though it was not strictly true. I also assured her that I would be going to the Bankks Club next Monday and would, therefore, see her then. She seemed reasonably happy to accept this arrangement and I felt that as there would be other people there I stood a reasonable chance of avoiding a difficult one-to-one situation with her.

CHAPTER THIRTY-ONE

Monday morning came around alarmingly quickly and I still had bad vibes about it. Although I hadn't got any patients booked in for a general anaesthetic and therefore my involvement in the morning's activities would be minimal, Spencer had asked me to be present so that I could familiarise myself with Dr MacKean's way of working. He was no doubt hoping that before long we would have a full morning of patients all lined up to experience the delights of being rendered unconscious for their treatment. I hadn't told him that unless my feelings on the subject changed very drastically, it was most unlikely that I would be playing a major part in it.

Spencer was in quite a flap when I arrived at the surgery. I think he was slightly apprehensive about the session and it showed in his behaviour. He was flitting from one thing to another without actually achieving anything, in a most disconcerting way and seemed very relieved when the doorbell rang and Balfour MacKean entered.

In spite of Spencer's eagerness to get organised for the session, Balfour announced that he couldn't even contemplate starting until he had had some coffee to spur him into action. Spencer was hoping that they could take their cups through to the surgery and drink whilst they were setting up but Balfour had a different idea. He sat down, with his coffee, in the chair in the office that was used for taking X-rays and proceeded to read his newspaper. He sipped the hot liquid far too slowly for Spencer, who was becoming quite agitated and finally could stand it no longer.

'I really think we ought to go and get this anaesthetic machine set up, Balfour. After all, you haven't used it before and you might need to get to know it before you use it on a patient.'

'As long as it's got gas in it, I should be able to figure it out,' Balfour replied without taking his eyes off his newspaper. 'I don't think there is a machine that I'm not familiar with. After all, there aren't that many different makes.'

I wasn't sure whether Balfour's nonchalance increased or reduced my uneasiness. Should I be encouraged by his apparent lack of concern, or was this display of indifference dangerous? I wasn't sure, but I can remember feeling even more relieved that I would only be a spectator.

After a good ten minutes, during which Spencer was pacing around and fiddling with odd bits of paper, Balfour folded up his paper and set his cup on the desk. 'Right, then, let's go and have a look at this gas machine.'

Spencer sprang after him and they both went through to the surgery, followed closely by myself, then Ingrid. Beryl stayed in the office typing.

'My God, Spencer, this is an ancient one,' were Balfour's first words when he saw the general anaesthetic machine. 'When was it last used?'

'I'm not really sure,' Spencer replied. 'My father used it from time to time. He used to give the gas and extract the teeth himself, as dentists did in those days. They didn't bother getting doctors in to help them, even though they hadn't received much training in general anaesthetics; in fact, they probably hadn't received any formal training. They just learnt on the job.'

'A rather dangerous way of doing things, I would say,' Balfour stated. 'I heard a rather tragic story the other day about a dentist who was giving a general anaesthetic to a patient. Apparently he didn't even have a nurse present; there was just him and the patient. Anyway, he put the patient to sleep and tried to extract a tooth. I can only think it was a particularly difficult extraction, as the poor dentist had a heart attack and died on the spot. Fortunately, the mask fell off the patient's face and he regained consciousness, but it must have been a hell of a shock to find the dentist slumped over him, dead. The patient was also quite upset that the dentist hadn't managed to complete the extraction before he died, and was quite put out to find that the offending tooth was still in his mouth.'

'That's terrible,' said Spencer, 'but I do think the dentist was foolish to give gas to a patient without there being anyone else present. The other thing you have to be careful about, of course, is if the patient is female you'll need to have a witness, in case you are accused of behaving improperly.'

All the time this conversation was going on Balfour was fiddling with the knobs and looking at the gauges. 'We need some halothane in the vaporiser. Have you got any?'

'Yes,' Spencer replied. 'I bought a new bottle; here it is. I found some in the cupboard, but as it was probably about fifteen years old I thought it might have lost its strength.'

'Good thinking, Spencer,' said Balfour pouring the liquid into the machine. 'I am not too sure about some of these rubber hoses. They look a bit perished to me, but the gas seems to be coming out of the mask, so with a bit of luck it should be all right. Has the patient arrived?'

'I'm not sure,' said Spencer. 'Will you go and see, please, Ingrid?'

'Yes, of course.'

She returned a few minutes later to confirm that Mr Dowland was in the waiting room and ready for his treatment.

'In that case, you may go and fetch him. I think we are ready.'

'Good morning, Mr Dowland. I am Dr MacKean, your anaesthetist. You know Mr Padginton, of course, and this is his assistant, Mr Derwent. Would you like to come and take a seat?'

Mr Dowland did as requested and Balfour took out his stethoscope. 'I need to listen to your heart before we begin, to make sure you are fit and healthy.'

Watching Balfour listening to Mr Dowland's heart brought back memories of my own medical examination with him, and I noticed with some amusement the same protrusion of his lower lip and the expansion of his jowls. Just as when he examined me, it took some considerable time before he was satisfied that Mr Dowland's heart was sound.

'Are you on any medication, Mr Dowland?'

'Not at present. I have been on painkillers and antibiotics for this tooth, but I finished them last week.'

'Good,' declared Balfour, 'and are you allergic to anything?'

'Not that I know of.'

'Good. Have you ever had a general anaesthetic before?'

'Not at the dentist, but I did in hospital when I had my appendix out.'

'Uh huh, and did you have any problems with the anaesthetic?'

'No, none at all. It all went very smoothly.'

'Good. Do you suffer with asthma or bronchitis?'

'No.'

'Good. Do you smoke?'

'No, I gave up ten years ago.'

'Good. Have you ever taken steroids?

'No I don't think so.'

'Good. Have you ever been on any medication which necessitated you carrying a card around with you?'

'Er, no.'

'Good. If you cut yourself, does it stop bleeding without any trouble?'

I could see that Spencer was becoming a little bit impatient with this extended interrogation and he intervened.

'You will see that there is a full medical history attached to his record card, Balfour.'

Balfour, however, refused to be put off. 'I prefer to do my own checks thank you, Spencer. Do you drink much beer, Mr Dowland?'

'Beer? I go to the pub four or five times a week and probably have three or four pints. Why is that important?'

'Well, in my experience heavy beer drinkers tend to resist the anaesthetic and we have to give them more to get them under. They can also kick and struggle in the early stages of the anaesthetic, so we like to be prepared for it.'

'I see but I'm not a heavy beer drinker, am I?'

'Moderately heavy, I would say, but now that we are aware of it we can take steps to compensate so there shouldn't be any trouble. Now is there someone with you to take you home in case you are a bit drowsy after the anaesthetic?'

'Yes, my wife is with me.'

'Fine, and just one last question. Have you had anything to eat or drink this morning?'

'Yes I had a good breakfast about an hour ago.'

I could see the look of utter despair come over Spencer's face and he could not contain his exasperation. 'You stupid man,' he cried out.

Mr Dowland looked bewildered. 'I thought I might not be able to eat after having a tooth out, so I thought I had better have a good feed before I came here. Have I done the wrong thing?'

Balfour remained expressionless but simply announced to the patient, 'I am afraid there is no way that we can proceed with this anaesthetic, Mr Dowland. Weren't you told that you must not have anything to eat or drink on the morning of the operation?'

'No, nobody said I couldn't eat.'

'I assumed that you would know that you shouldn't eat anything before a general anaesthetic. Everybody knows that,' shouted Spencer.

'One should never assume anything,' said Balfour, looking superciliously at Spencer over the top of his spectacles, which had slipped to the end of his nose. 'I always think it is a good idea to give the patient a printed sheet of instructions, and then everyone knows where they stand.'

Spencer didn't reply but was obviously seething inwardly at his own senselessness, as well as what he perceived to be stupidity on the part of Mr Dowland.

'I'd better go then,' declared Mr Dowland, sensing Spencer's hostility. He jumped out of the chair and was out of the door before anyone had time to say anything to him. He didn't ask about making another appointment.

'It would appear,' said Balfour, 'unless you have any other patients, the session has come to an end. I must admit though, Spencer, I am a bit concerned about this anaesthetic machine. I think there might be a bit of a leak on some of the connections and I suggest that you get it properly checked out and overhauled before the next session – if you intend to have one, that is.'

'Why yes, most certainly. I was thinking that we could perhaps arrange one in about a month, and that would give us time to find some patients to fill it.'

'As you wish,' said Balfour. 'If you phone through to my surgery with some suggested dates, I will see when I am free. Now gentlemen, I will wish you a very good morning and leave you to get on with your work.'

As he stood up he took out an envelope from his pocket and handed it to Spencer. 'Here is my account for the session. It is more or less what we agreed, except that we talked about a sessional fee of around twenty five pounds. I always feel it is more fitting for professionals to deal in guineas, I am sure you will agree, so I have made out the bill for twenty five guineas. Don't feel you have to settle it this very moment.'

'What a cheek,' said Spencer as soon as Balfour was out of the room. 'He didn't do anything, I earned nothing and it has cost me twenty five guineas.'

'It wasn't his fault that we didn't have any patients for him, and he has given up his morning,' I replied, trying to see it from both points of view. 'I didn't book any patients in either. You asked me to keep it clear so that I could see you and Balfour at work, so I didn't earn anything for myself or for the practice.'

'I know, I know,' was Spencer's irritated response. 'It has been a disastrous morning all round. As we both appear to be free now until lunchtime I am going to take the opportunity of going to the bank and doing some shopping. If you want something to do, Justin, have a look at the gas machine and find out which, if any of the pipes and connections need renewing and I'll see if I can track down some replacements. I don't see why I should pay an engineer to overhaul the machine if we can do it ourselves. It can't be that complicated. I'll be back later.'

Spencer departed and Ingrid joined Beryl in the office in order to catch up on some paperwork. Because there were no patients on the premises, Mrs Duck seized the opportunity to do some extra cleaning. Normally she would have gone home by now, but such was her dedication to her work that she was happy to stay on a bit longer.

I fetched a pair of pliers and a screwdriver from the boot of my car and set about inspecting the pipes of the anaesthetic machine. I didn't know very much about it but I thought it would be a simple enough matter to establish whether the rubber pipes were perished and if the connections were tight. How though, could I determine whether or not there were any leaks? When I turned the tap on, the noise of the gas hissing out of the facemask made it difficult to hear if it was hissing out from anywhere else. I put my hand around the connection to see if I could feel it on my skin; but I felt nothing. I thought that perhaps if I put my ear close to the connection I might be able to hear gas escaping. I did this on each of the connections, though some of them were difficult to reach and called for major contortions of the head and neck in order to get close enough. Also, when attempting this, I overlooked the fact that when my ear was close to the point of escape, my nose wasn't far away from it either.

Mrs Duck had been in and out of the surgery several times with her duster and vacuum cleaner, but when she entered this time she received an awful shock. She dropped her tin of polish, let out a scream and ran back to the office where Beryl and Ingrid were working.

'It's Justin,' she cried out. 'He's lying on the floor in a pool of blood. I think he's dead.'

CHAPTER THIRTY-TWO

Ingrid and Beryl jumped up from their chairs in horror and ran into Spencer's surgery to find me lying on the floor. When I fell down, the back of my head had struck the sharp edge of Spencer's metal foot pedal making a deep cut which was pouring blood over my hair, operating coat and the linoleum surface that Mrs Duck had just polished.

'Justin, can you hear me?' Beryl shouted. 'Go and phone for an ambulance, Ingrid, quickly. Justin, can you hear me?'

Slowly I regained consciousness to see a very blurred image of Beryl bending over me. I was immediately aware of a dull ache at the back of my head, which steadily increased to a severe throbbing. Beryl placed a sterile dressing over it to catch the blood.

'Don't try to move, Justin, help is on the way,' said Beryl comfortingly.

'I'll be all right,' I replied, valiantly trying to sit up. I began to realise what had happened and I couldn't help feeling foolish that I hadn't treated the anaesthetic machine with more respect. I should have remembered that it contained powerful agents designed to render someone unconscious and that if I stuck my nose close enough to inhale the gases that's what would happen to me.

'I'm fine.'

'You are not fine. You have a nasty cut on the back of your head that will need looking at. Ingrid has phoned for an ambulance.'

Ingrid came in. 'The ambulance is on its way. Thank goodness you are conscious, Justin, Mrs Duck thought you were dead.'

'Not quite, though I do feel like death warmed up.' Again I tried to get up and this time I resisted Beryl's attempts to stop me. 'I can't lie here all morning. I'll be all right sitting up.'

The ambulance arrived very quickly and soon I was carried, in spite of my assertions that I was perfectly capable of walking, down the stairs and out to the waiting vehicle. Several people had gathered round to watch, and I hoped that none of them would be patients of mine.

As my mind threw off the effects of the gas, I felt more and more stupid about the entire episode and more and more pain from the gash on my head. The ambulance sped on its way to the casualty department of the nearest hospital and one of the members of the two-man crew looked at my wound.

'It's a nasty cut, old son. It will need a few stitches. How did it happen?'

'I was trying to repair our general anaesthetic machine and was overcome by the gas. When I fell down, I must have banged my head on a metal foot pedal. At least I didn't feel anything at the time, because I was anaesthetised.'

'Oh yes? I've heard about dentists having a quick whiff of the gas. Some of them get addicted to it, don't they?'

'I don't know but I can assure you that I'm not addicted to it, and if I had intended having a therapeutic whiff of it I wouldn't have done it standing up; I would have sat down first. As a matter of fact, this was the first time we have ever used the gas machine since I joined the practice. My boss went on a course in London and came back with the bright idea of doing gas sessions, so he dug out this old machine from the loft. It's donkey's years old and leaks gas from some of the connections. I was trying to find the source of the leaks and next thing I knew I was lying on my back on the floor.'

'Very nasty. It seems to me it would be safer to entrust the repair of the machine to the professionals.'

'Personally, I'd be much happier to see it dumped completely. I had a bad feeling about the idea of doing general anaesthetics from the moment my boss suggested it, but it was the poor patients I was worried about. I never thought I would be the one to come to grief.'

'Don't worry, they'll soon have you sorted. We are at the hospital now.'

I was allowed to walk, with assistance, from the ambulance and once inside I was told to lie on a trolley. After about ten minutes I was taken through to a treatment room and ten stitches were inserted into my scalp. I was foolish enough to think that once this was done I would be able to leave.

'I want you to have an X-ray to check that there aren't any skull fractures,' said the consultant. 'We will wheel you out into the corridor and they will come and fetch you when they are ready. I'll look at the X-ray as soon as it's available, and then we'll take it from there.'

It was about three quarters of an hour before I was wheeled to radiography. I wondered how long it would take to get the X-ray developed, as I was already becoming impatient to get out of the hospital. I can't say how long it took to develop the film, but it was almost two hours before I saw the consultant again.

'I can't see a fracture on the X-ray, Mr Derwent, but I wonder if perhaps it would be advisable for us to keep you in overnight, checking on you every hour to make sure there aren't any complications.'

'Surely that isn't necessary?' I protested. 'Apart from a bit of a headache I feel fine. I'm sure it's just a cut, and now that you have stitched it up it will be all right.'

'Hopefully it will, but it's best not to take any chances. Will there be someone with you at home to keep an eye on you?'

Foolishly I replied, 'no, I live alone.'

'In that case, I insist that you stay here where we can monitor your progress. Lie there and take it easy and we'll sort out a bed for you.'

Lying on a trolley in a hospital corridor is not my idea of a pleasant way to spend a day, but it seemed I didn't have much choice. It was almost five o'clock by the time I was finally transported to a ward, presented with a pair of hospital pyjamas and told to get into bed. The thing that struck me first about the ward was the intense heat. Admittedly I lived in a draughty old cottage with little or no heating, so most places were going to be warm by comparison, but this was ridiculous. Surely nobody felt comfortable at that temperature. Sweat poured off me and I began to think I was running a fever, but the hourly checks of my pulse, blood pressure, temperature and reflexes had so far failed to reveal any abnormality. I asked one of the nurses if it might be possible to open a window but the suggestion was stamped upon immediately on the grounds that it carried far too great a risk of some patients catching cold. My view was that without fresh air and with that degree of heat, the ward was a breeding ground for infection, which actually increased the chances of catching something. However, it was futile to try and argue with the nurse about it; she was obviously just obeying rules.

At least I thought it would soon be time for the evening meal. I hadn't had so much as a cup of tea since breakfast, and I was starving. I had heard that hospital food could be fairly basic and I knew I couldn't exactly expect cordon bleu cooking, but I was so hungry I didn't care; I could have eaten virtually anything. Unfortunately, I was in for another unpleasant shock.

'I am afraid we have to keep you empty, Mr Derwent,' came the shattering announcement from the nurse, 'in case we have to give you an anaesthetic to operate on you. You may sip some water, but that's all.'

I was incredulous. Although my headache was not improving, I was convinced that there was no reason at all why I should not go home. To be told that I would not be getting any food was just too much for me to bear, but what could I do? I had heard of people discharging themselves from hospital, but I didn't have the strength of character to be that assertive, so I had no alternative but to lie in bed sweating and watching the clock go round.

Just after six o'clock, Ingrid and Spencer came to see me.

'Hello, Justin. You look much better now than you did this morning when the ambulance took you away,' said Ingrid. 'I was so worried about you.'

'Thanks for your concern and for coming to visit me, Ingrid. I am very pleased to see you.'

'I have brought you a photographic magazine. I thought you might need something to read.'

'Thank you, Ingrid, that was very thoughtful of you.'

Spencer was less sympathetic. 'That was a damn silly thing to do if you don't mind my saying so, Justin. How on earth did it happen?'

'I was trying to find the gas leak on your anaesthetic machine, and the next thing I know I'm on the floor.'

'Did you find where the gas was coming from?' asked Spencer somewhat insensitively.

'I'm afraid not. I passed out before I got that far.'

'Pity,' said Spencer. 'We need to get it sorted out before our next gas session in four weeks' time.'

'You'll forgive me if I have nothing more to do with it.'

'I don't blame you for not wanting to be involved,' said Ingrid. 'The machine is dangerous. But forget the silly machine, I am sure you don't want to think about it any more. Are they looking after you in here?'

'They have stitched up my head but unfortunately they won't feed me in case I have to have an operation and an anaesthetic.'

Spencer burst out laughing. 'I'm sorry, Justin, but it struck me as amusing that you gave yourself an anaesthetic this morning and it didn't seem to matter then that you had eaten breakfast. Perhaps the importance of fasting before an anaesthetic is overrated.'

'Balfour seemed to think it was important with Mr Dowland,' I replied.

'What a disaster. The stupid man should have known not to tuck into a hearty breakfast before having a G.A. He wasted everybody's time. I'm going to get some instructions printed up as Balfour suggested to avoid the same thing happening again.'

'It sounds a good idea if you are convinced about continuing with gas sessions.'

'Oh, absolutely,' Spencer enthused. 'I am sure it could be very profitable for the practice.'

'The first one wasn't very profitable, was it?' I replied sarcastically. 'You finished up out of pocket on that one.'

'I know. We shouldn't have arranged it so soon. We needed more time to fill the session, but it will be all right next time.'

He paused and adopted a more serious attitude. 'Oh, by the way, what's this about you refusing to make Mrs Johnson a crown before she went on holiday? After she saw you she went home and wrote a letter to me. She was obviously very upset at the way you treated her.'

'She had broken a crown. I said that I would fit her with a temporary, but there wasn't time to make a permanent

266

replacement for her as we only had two days before she flew off to New Zealand.'

'You can easily get a crown made in two days. Melvyn has often done it for me. In fact, I got one made for Mrs Johnson in two days quite recently. She is a private patient, Justin, or was. She may well have left the practice now, thanks to you. We must always be prepared to put ourselves out to please private patients because they form the backbone of our practice. I can't imagine what made you refuse to do it for her.'

'But you said to me that I must never, never allow myself to deviate from our normal procedure in order to fulfil patients' wishes and demands. You also said that it was a golden rule that you yourself always followed. You told me that the day before you went to London. I would have got a crown made for her, but felt I had to follow your instructions.'

'That's nonsense, Justin. I would never turn away a private patient, especially a long-standing one, who was prepared to pay over the odds because it was an emergency. You must never do that again, Justin, do I make myself clear?'

I felt utterly puzzled by Spencer's outburst. There was total inconsistency in what he had said to me, and I felt I wanted to discuss the matter further in an attempt to clarify the position for the future but Ingrid intervened.

'I don't think you should be talking to Justin about this matter at the moment, Spencer. He had a nasty experience today and needs to rest. You mustn't upset him. You can take this up with him when he gets back to the surgery, but this is not the time or the place.'

Ingrid sounded very authoritative in spite of her youth and Spencer didn't try to overrule her.

'Are they likely to let you go home tomorrow?' he asked.

'I sincerely hope so. I don't want to stay here a moment longer than I have to. It's so hot.'

'It is warm in here,' agreed Ingrid. Spencer, however, was more concerned about when I would be back at work.

'We'll cancel your patients for tomorrow but we'll leave Wednesday as it stands at the moment. Hopefully you will be back at work then.'

'For goodness sake, show a bit more sympathy, Spencer,' said Ingrid. 'Justin might need the rest of the week to get over this. I don't think you should pressurise him to return to work before he is ready.'

'No, no, of course not,' said Spencer. 'Ingrid is quite right. Take as long as you need and don't come back to work until you are ready. All I meant was that we can take it one day at a time; we won't cancel your Wednesday patients just yet, in case you feel well enough to come back.'

'I should be all right by Wednesday. I shall feel better when I get something to eat, and considerably better once I am told I can go home.'

Ingrid and Spencer stayed with me for almost an hour and after they had left I felt very restless once again. I wasn't allowed to get out of bed and every hour without fail a nurse arrived to check that I wasn't taking a turn for the worse as a result of my accident.

At eight o'clock all of the other patients' visitors, some of whom had been there for the whole of the permitted four hours from four until eight, were asked to leave the ward and everything began to shut down for the night. I had heard that in hospital the day starts early, I now found out that it also finishes early.

I was reading the magazine Ingrid had brought for me, as eight o'clock was a little early for me to go to sleep, even if it had been a trying day. At around eight fifteen, a nurse came to my bed and said, 'Mr Derwent, your fiancée is here and desperately wants to see you.'

'My what?' I exclaimed.

'Your fiancée. She knows that visiting ends at eight o'clock and she is deeply apologetic for being late, but she was unavoidably detained and has begged us to let her see you for a few moments. She is very distressed, and Sister thought that as it's your fiancée, in the circumstances she might let you have just a short time together, but we wanted to check that you weren't asleep before we agreed. Would you like me to show her in?'

I guessed immediately that it would be Annette and I very nearly told the nurse that she wasn't my fiancée, but then I thought that it might be better if I didn't. First of all it would create a difficult situation for Annette, which would have been churlish of me after she had taken the trouble to come and see me. In any event, and in spite of her presumptuousness, I was pleased to have someone to talk to and alleviate the boredom, if only for a few minutes.

'Yes, show her in,' I replied.

'Justin, my darling, are you all right,' cried Annette throwing her arms around me and kissing me passionately on the lips. There were tears in her eyes.

'I'm fine, thanks Annette. Thank you for coming to see me. What's all this about being my fiancée?'

'I'm sorry I had to say that, but I didn't think they would let me in if I said I was just a friend. I do hope you don't mind. I had to come and see you. I was devastated when I heard what happened to you.'

'How did you find out?'

'When you didn't turn up at the Bankks Club this evening I knew something must have happened to you because you told me you would be there. I tried phoning you at home but of course there was no reply, so I phoned your practice to see if they knew where you were. I think it was your boss's wife I spoke to. She told me about your accident at work this morning and that you had been taken to hospital. I hear that you cut your head very badly.'

'It was a little cut that needed a few stitches, but apart from being very sore it isn't too bad.'

'Let me see it.'

I lifted my head off the pillow so that Annette could see the wound.

'Oh Justin, it looks very painful. It must be bad or they wouldn't have kept you in.'

'They just want to make sure there aren't any complications and they were worried because I live alone.'

'I would have come and stayed with you and looked after you, Justin. You only had to phone me and I would have come straight away.'

'That's very sweet of you, Annette, but there really was no need. Hopefully they will let me go home first thing tomorrow morning.'

'Will you phone me and let me know as soon as they say you can go home? I will come and fetch you if you want me to.'

'You don't need to do that, Annette, but thanks for the offer.'

Much to Annette's dismay, the nurse came to my bedside. 'I'm afraid I must ask you to leave now.'

Annette looked disappointed but didn't object. 'Yes, of course,' she replied. 'Thank you for letting me see him. Goodnight, darling. I shall be thinking of you every minute of the night and tomorrow until I see you again.'

She put her arms round me once again and gave me another kiss. I felt that I had to go along with the pretence for the nurse's benefit, so I tried my best to look as if I were kissing my fiancée but at the same time I hoped I wouldn't be raising hopes in Annette's mind that weren't really justified.

CHAPTER THIRTY-THREE

I wondered why the day had to begin quite so early for patients in hospital. It seemed to me that the days there were long and boring enough without starting them at some ungodly hour. At six o'clock the nurses went round to wake up all the patients and told all those who were able to do so to go and have a wash.

As I had been woken up every hour throughout the night to check on my condition, I was by now well beyond the point of trying to sleep any more; I was wide awake. Although my health was not giving any cause for concern, I wasn't allowed the privilege of performing my own ablutions, nor was I given any breakfast.

'You must stay in bed at the moment, Mr Derwent, and we can't feed you until the doctor has seen you and given his permission. He will be coming to see you when he does his rounds today and I should think you will then be allowed to go home.'

The nurse's words sounded good. I couldn't wait.

'Do you know what time that will be?'

'I don't, I'm afraid. It depends who is on duty and whether there are any emergencies for him to deal with.'

With any luck, I thought, I might be home by lunchtime. I didn't know at what time doctors did their rounds but I imagined it would be between ten and eleven o'clock. I don't know why I thought that, but it just seemed likely that it would be at that sort of time. I was sure that my injury was no more than a nasty cut and as that had now been dealt with and there were no complications, the doctor would have no hesitation in discharging me. All I could do was to wait for him to come and see me.

I continued to read the magazine Ingrid had given to me; after all, it was the only thing I had to read. I read every page thoroughly and slowly in an attempt to make it last as long as possible, though I hoped that I would be seen by the doctor before I got to the end of it.

I hadn't been reading very long when two young nurses presented themselves at my bedside.

'We have come to give you a wash, Mr Derwent, and to make sure you aren't getting bedsores.'

'Bedsores! I have only been here one night. I'm hardly likely to be developing bedsores just yet. And in any case, I am perfectly capable of taking myself for a wash, thank you very much.'

'Until the doctor has seen you, you can't get out of bed so we have to wash you and all patients are checked for bedsores every morning. It doesn't matter whether you have been here one day or one year. Now, please unbutton your pyjama trousers and turn over on to your tummy.'

'I reluctantly did as I was asked and a further wave of humiliation washed over me. I was relieved that the nurses were swift and highly professional in carrying out their duties and soon I was allowed to return to my magazine.

As they left me to move on to the next patient I said, 'Am I allowed to go to the toilet?'

'I'm afraid not; you must use a bedpan. Would you like me to get one for you?'

'No, I can wait until after the doctor has seen me. Has he started his rounds yet?'

'I don't think so, it's a bit early at the moment. Doctor Badger who is in charge of you rarely starts before eleven o'clock, and sometimes it is much later than that.'

'How much later?' I demanded, desperately hoping it wouldn't be.

'It's difficult to say. He will probably see you late morning but just occasionally he gets delayed and he doesn't get round until sometime after lunch.'

'Which I won't be eating!'

'That's right. Not unless he has been to see you first.'

I groaned with despair.

I had never in my life known time pass so slowly. It was unbelievable that the clock always ticked along at the same speed, and yet sometimes it seemed to be at a snail's pace and at other times it was like lightning. When I took exams, time always seemed to pass more quickly than at any other time I could think of, except of course when one was asleep. If only I could sleep, that would be the best solution to my boredom but I simply wasn't tired or I was too keyed up to sleep, and in any case I was still having my blood pressure checked every hour. I tried to think of ways to make the time pass more quickly but I failed miserably. I read my magazine from cover to cover, over and over again and every time I heard footsteps in the corridor I gazed in eager anticipation at the door, hoping that it would be Dr Badger starting his rounds.

Little by little the morning dragged along. Lunchtime arrived and I had to suffer the added torture of watching the other patients eat whilst all I could do was to lie there sipping water. I was by now thinking that the whole thing was becoming quite ridiculous. I was obviously going to be all right, so why was my agony being prolonged in this way? I thought hospitals were short of beds. Surely it would be best for everyone if they were shot of me.

Dr Badger finally arrived at my bedside around half past three. He seemed to materialise from nowhere and deprived me of the satisfaction of seeing him enter through the door I had been watching so assiduously all morning. He looked at my notes, which were hanging on the foot of my bed and made a cursory examination of the cut on the back of my head.

'You will need to go and see your own GP in a week's time to get the stitches removed, but I see no reason why you shouldn't go home now.'

The words came like a reprieve from a sentence of death. I was ready to leap out of bed, dressing myself as I ran down the stairs, such was my haste to get out of there. The nurse, however, sensed my impatience and moderated my impetuousness.

'I would take it a bit steady if I were you. You might feel a bit weak when you get out of bed. Don't forget you haven't eaten anything for over twenty-four hours. I'll pull the curtains around your bed so you can get dressed, but take it slowly and sit down if you feel faint. I'll go and fetch you a cup of tea and a sandwich which I think you ought to have before you leave.'

'Thank you,' I replied though I wasn't anxious to prolong my stay any longer than was absolutely necessary. When my feet touched the floor, however, I understood what she meant as I immediately began to feel distinctly queasy. Dressing took considerably longer than I had anticipated and I had to keep sitting down.

'I see what you mean,' I admitted to her when she returned with my tea and a cheese sandwich. My pallid face told her how I was feeling.

'Sit down and eat this slowly. We don't want you falling down and hurting yourself again, do we? You will soon feel stronger, but you need to take it easy for a while.'

I suddenly became aware that my unfortunate accident had had a much greater effect upon me than I realised and that it might take a few days for me to get over it. Although I had been desperately hungry for most of the time I was lying in bed, now my appetite had deserted me. I sipped the warm tea and took tiny bites of the sandwich which I turned over and over in my mouth before I was able to swallow them. I felt as if the stuffing had been knocked out of me completely and I sat there feeling thoroughly sorry for myself.

My drifting thoughts were abruptly pulled back into line by a female voice behind me.

'I've come to take you home, Justin.'

I swung round expecting to see the dark hair and brown eyes of Annette, but I didn't. Instead I saw blue eyes and blonde hair. It was Sarah.

'Sarah,' I exclaimed in amazement, 'How lovely to see you.'

'Hello, Justin. How are you feeling?'

'A bit weak, but I shall be fine when I get home. I haven't eaten since yesterday's breakfast and I'm not good if I don't get food. How did you know I was here?'

'I telephoned your surgery today. I only got back from Kent yesterday evening and I was going to phone you at home, but I realised it was Monday so I thought you would be at the Bankks Club. I didn't get back early enough to go there myself. I was horrified to hear what you had done. How on earth did it happen?'

'I feel so stupid about it. I was trying to repair my boss's ancient gas machine and unfortunately I gassed myself. That in itself wouldn't have been too bad but I managed to cut my head when I fell down.'

'Ouch, that looks sore,' Sarah exclaimed, looking at my stitched wound. 'Finish your tea and I will drive you straight home.'

'That's very kind of you, Sarah, but I don't want you to go to any trouble. I can always get a taxi.'

'It's no trouble at all, Justin. I came here thinking you might want a lift home.'

'Are you back from Kent for good now?'

'Yes. Hopefully my mother and I have tied up all the loose ends and sorted out our affairs so we can start a new life here. I'm really looking forward to it.'

'Kent is nice, isn't it?'

'It is, but I feel a bit cut off there. You are out on a limb a little bit and it's an awful bind having to get round London every time you want to go somewhere else in the country.'

'Don't you have friends there you will be sad to leave?'

'Not very many. Most of them have moved away for one reason or another. There isn't really anyone special.'

'I'm surprised you aren't leaving a boyfriend behind, an attractive girl like you.'

Sarah blushed slightly. 'There was someone once but that ended a long time ago and we have both moved on. There hasn't been anyone else since.'

'Does he still live in Kent?'

'Yes I think so, but I haven't seen him for over a year. As I said, it is all over and I am quite happy about it. The relationship just sort of fizzled out and I wouldn't want to resurrect it. Anyway that's enough about my past. Let's get you home.'

'My car is still parked outside the surgery, or I hope it is.'

'We can pick that up later. At the moment I think you should go home and take it easy. I will prepare you something more substantial to eat. You will probably feel a lot better if you can get some food inside you.'

'That's very kind of you, Sarah.'

'Not at all, Justin. I am more than happy to do it. After all, that's what friends are for.'

CHAPTER THIRTY-FOUR

I began to feel somewhat better once I was outside the hospital. I don't think the heat of the ward really suited me and the coolness of the light breeze on my face was wonderfully refreshing. With every step I took, my queasiness gradually diminished and by the time we had reached Sarah's car which was parked about three hundred yards away in the hospital car park, I felt almost back to normal. Only the dull throbbing pain at the back of my head persisted to remind me of yesterday's unfortunate incident.

'We are virtually going right past the door of my practice. I could pick up my car on the way,' I said to Sarah as I climbed into the passenger seat of her red Mini Minor.

'Are you sure you are well enough, Justin? I can always run you back for it later.'

'I'm all right. I don't like to leave it there, really. Being a soft top, anyone can break into it. It was left outside on the road all last night and I don't want to leave it there any longer. I imagine Spencer would have let me know if anything happened to it, but I would be much happier if it were at home in the garage.'

'As long as you're sure you will be all right. I'll drop you off at your practice, then follow you back to your house.'

I was very relieved to find my car safe. It instantly roared into life as soon as I pressed the starter switch and soon I had it safely locked away in the garage.

'You live in a lovely little house,' said Sarah looking at the diminutive old cottage which looked particularly attractive in its woodland setting with the surrounding trees casting flickering shadows on to the rough stone walls.

'Yes, it is nice.'

'I would love to live in a house like this.'

'It's a bit cold in winter.'

'I wouldn't mind that. It can be pretty cold in Kent, and we lived in a draughty old house which never really got warm, so I'm used to it. The house didn't have as much character as yours, though.'

'It isn't really mine. I only rent it.'

'You were lucky to find somewhere as nice as this to rent. There aren't that many rental properties about. My mother and I are renting at the moment until she finds something she wants to buy, but it isn't as exciting as this little place.'

'Come inside and I'll show you round.'

No sooner had we stepped inside the door when the phone rang. It was Spencer, sounding extremely agitated about something.

'Oh, there you are, Justin. I phoned the hospital and they told me you had left with a young lady who was taking you home. I don't quite know how to tell you this, but I am afraid it looks as if your car has been stolen. I popped out to the shops a little while ago and it was outside the practice when I left, but when I got back it had gone. Neither Ingrid nor Beryl saw anyone drive off in it. It just seems that one minute it was there and the next minute it had gone. I am so sorry to have to break the news to you. I know how much that car means to you.'

Spencer was genuinely concerned and I received the impression that to some extent he felt guilty about not having kept a closer watch on it. My first reaction was to string him along and not say that I had collected it myself but I decided against it.

'It's all right, Spencer. My friend, Sarah, picked me up from the hospital and dropped me off at the practice. I drove the car home.'

'You mean you drove it away without telling anyone at the practice? We have been beside ourselves with worry here. I've had a sleepless night looking out of the window every few minutes to make sure it was still there. You could have let us know you were moving it.'

Now it was my turn to feel guilty.

'I'm sorry, Spencer, I didn't think. I can see now that I should have called in at the surgery to tell someone, but I was anxious to get home,'

'Couldn't wait to get back to your place with your friend. Sarah, no doubt. So, who is this one? We haven't heard anything about her.'

'Just a friend. I met her for the first time a few weeks ago, but then she had to go back to Kent with her mother and only got back here yesterday.'

'I see. Well, obviously your judgement was clouded by this young woman's presence, but it would have been nice if you had let us know you were moving the car instead of letting us all think it had been stolen.'

'I really am sorry, Spencer.'

'Okay. Apology accepted. Are you going to come back to work tomorrow, or shall we start cancelling your patients?'

'I'll be there.'

'Are you sure you are well enough to come back?'

'Yes, I'm fine.'

'That's good then. I look forward to seeing you back in harness first thing tomorrow morning.'

'Goodbye, Spencer.'

'I'll put the kettle on,' exclaimed Sarah. 'I expect you could do with a cup of tea, then I'll see about getting you something to eat.'

'I think I need something stronger than tea. How about a whisky?'

'As you haven't eaten anything since yesterday morning except for a cheese sandwich, I don't think that is a very good idea,' Sarah replied.

'You haven't come here to boss me about, have you?' I replied smiling.

'No, I have come here to take care of you. I have your best interests at heart. You can have a whisky if you want one. I merely said that I didn't think it was a very good idea on a stomach as empty as yours.'

'You are probably right, Sarah, and I do appreciate your fetching me from the hospital.'

'It's a pleasure, Justin. Now you sit down and take it easy, and I'll see what I can rustle up for you to eat.'

'I think you might find it difficult if you are relying on what's in the fridge. It's practically empty.'

'You men are hopeless on your own. It's a bad sign that you haven't any food in the house but you've got whisky.'

Sarah looked in the fridge and larder and decided that it would be virtually impossible to put together anything vaguely resembling even a light snack.

'You stay here and drink your tea,' she announced. 'I'll go and get us some food. I won't be long.'

Sarah took a long drink from her cup and left to go to the shops. I went into my sitting room and sat down on the sofa thinking that it was good to be back home. That was the first time I had been in hospital and frankly I wasn't enamoured with it. I hoped sincerely that I would never have to go in ever again.

Lack of sleep had left me feeling quite tired and soon I began to drift. My peace was short lived, however, as suddenly there was a hammering on the door so violent I was surprised it wasn't knocked off its hinges. I jumped up out of the chair and, thinking that the call must be extremely urgent, I ran to the door and opened it as quickly as I could. As soon as the lock was released, the door flew open with the force of half a dozen horses. I was pushed out of the way and almost trampled underfoot as Annette shot through like a bolt of lightning.

'Sarah's here, isn't she?' she demanded.

'No she isn't,' I uttered unconvincingly, completely stunned by her outburst.

'Yes she is,' Annette insisted. 'Where is she?'

Before I could say any more she ran into the kitchen, then she turned and pushed me out of the way once again and mounted the stairs three treads at a time. By the time I had followed her upstairs she had been in both bedrooms and the bathroom.

'She must be hiding. I know she's here.'

'What makes you think that, Annette? You have seen for yourself that she isn't.'

'I called in at your practice on the way here less than ten minutes ago and your boss told me you were with Sarah. How could you do it to me, Justin? You know how I feel about you.'

'I haven't done anything,' I protested. 'I was getting ready to leave hospital and Sarah turned up and offered to take me home, that's all.'

'We had arranged for me to pick you up and take you home.'

'I wasn't aware that we made a definite arrangement and as Sarah was there I saw no reason not to go with her.'

'Why did she go to the hospital anyway? Have you been in touch with her? You have, haven't you? You have been in touch with her secretly all along. How could you, Justin? I didn't think you were like that.'

'I haven't been in touch with her at all. I haven't spoken to her or heard anything from her since the first evening I went to the Bankks Club. Apparently she came back from Kent on Monday and found out on Tuesday that I was in hospital, and she just turned up there out of the blue as I was about to leave. That's all there is to it.'

'She must be hiding,' insisted Annette. 'Where is she?'

'She has gone to get us some food because I didn't have anything in the house to eat.'

'I wanted to be the one to pick you up from the hospital and to take you home and look after you. I thought that's what you wanted too.'

'I'm sorry, Annette, I didn't think about it.'

'Well, isn't that what you want? Don't you want me be around to look after you?'

'It's very kind of you to want to help but ...'

'I'm not doing it to be kind. I'm doing it to show you how I feel for you. Don't you feel the same way about me?'

'I look upon you as a very good friend – a lovely friend – but I would be deceiving you if I said there was any more to it than that.'

I had tried to choose my words carefully but somehow I don't think I got it quite right as Annette immediately burst into floods of tears.

'I thought we had a future together,' she sobbed. 'I felt sure that you had strong feelings for me. The day we went out to Tom's boat you were so gentle and, and loving towards me.'

'You were upset about your fiancé letting you down on your wedding day and I tried to comfort you, that's all.'

'That's all? That's all?' Annette screamed.

There were more floods of tears and she turned and fled from the cottage. She went so fast I would have found it difficult to catch her even if I had tried. Frankly, I didn't know what to do. I had been aware that her feelings had been running away with her and I had tried to calm things down, but clearly I hadn't made a very good job of it. I hated to think that I had hurt her but it had certainly not been intentional, and in any event, it was surely best for her to know the truth even if it was painful. I liked Annette; she was a sweet girl and didn't deserve to be hurt in the way she had been in the past. I felt very sorry for her but I had to admit that my feelings for her were not what she was hoping for.

I sat down on my sofa feeling very upset. I didn't want to snub her, nor did I want our friendship to end, but I couldn't pretend that I wanted more than friendship and it would have been wrong of me to do so. I decided that the best course of action would be to leave her alone at the moment to let her calm down and make contact in a day or two to talk things through. I was still wondering about it when Sarah came back.

'Are you all right, Justin?' she asked, sensing that I had something on my mind.

'Yes, I'm all right. It's just that whilst you were out, Annette came round here like a mad woman, in a real state because she thought you were here.'

'Annette? Why should she be concerned about me being here?'

'She seems to have got it into her head that she and I might be an item.'

'Well are you or aren't you? Are you going out together?'

'No, not like that. She asked me to take her to her work's dinner because she didn't have anyone else to go with, but that's all.'

'Well then, if that's all, you are surely free to be with whoever you want. Aren't you?'

'Yes, I suppose so. It's just that I think Annette was hoping there might be more to our relationship than just friendship.'

'And you don't want more?'

'That's about right, but I do feel very sorry for her. Do you know anything about her past?'

'I know she was jilted at the altar, if that's what you mean.'

'Oh, you do know? I wasn't sure whether she had told you.'

'Yes, she told me the first time I met her. Understandably it had a strong impact upon her, but instead of it making her more wary of men it seems to have made her more desperate to find a replacement husband before it's too late.'

'Is that how you see it?' I asked, slightly shocked by what I thought was a somewhat harsh appraisal.

'I think that sums it up fairly accurately. If you want my honest opinion, I don't think she is too stable emotionally and frankly, if I were a man I would be very wary of getting involved with her. I think that once she gets her claws into someone she isn't going to give him an inch of breathing space for fear of losing him like she lost the last one.'

'All the same, I didn't want to hurt her.'

'You can't help it if you don't reciprocate her feelings. It's better she finds out sooner rather than later.'

'I suppose you are right. In fact, I know you are right. I am of the same opinion which is why I didn't want to lead her on but I can't help feeling a bit sorry for her.'

'I am sure she will get over it and find some other handsome young man. Now, this handsome young man needs to get some food inside him so sit down and I will serve it up for you.'

'Yes ma'am, whatever you say.'

Sarah had bought some cooked chicken, and served with salad and freshly baked bread. It tasted delicious and soon had me feeling more like my old self. She had also bought a bottle of white wine which had been chilled by the shop, and this was a perfect accompaniment to the meal.

Afterwards we sat down on the sofa together and listened to Rimsky-Korsakov's Scheherazade. It was one of those rare occasions when everything seemed just right. It was warm and comfortable in my small sitting room and utterly and completely peaceful. It came as a great disappointment to me when the record ended but the silence that followed accentuated the tranquillity in my little cottage.

Neither of us spoke for some moments then Sarah said, 'Isn't it peaceful here? All you can hear is the birds. We could be miles away from civilisation.'

'It is extremely quiet. It makes a very pleasant change from the bed sitting room I had when I was a student. That was only two minutes' walk away from the city centre and the noise of the traffic never stopped, day or night.'

'I'm really glad to be back here, you know, Justin. I didn't like Kent very much. I don't really know why, but somehow I never really took to it. Strangely enough, I feel completely at home in Dorset already, even though I have only been here a relatively short time. Perhaps the people I have met have had something to do with it.'

'I like it here. I wasn't sure whether I would settle. I thought I might find it too quiet after living in a busy city for six years, but I too feel very much at home now.'

I felt quite contented and the pain at the back of my head had more or less subsided, though the cut was still very tender if I rested that part of my head against the back of the chair. The events of the past twenty four hours were, however, beginning to catch up with me and suddenly I began to feel distinctly drowsy. I tried to hide it from Sarah but she seemed to spot it immediately.

'I have very much enjoyed being with you and listening to music', she said. 'I see we share the same taste. However, I think I ought to go home now and let you get some sleep. You must be absolutely worn out after your ordeal. I don't suppose you got much sleep in hospital and you need an early night, especially if you are going in to work tomorrow, though personally I think you ought to stay at home and rest.'

'I'll be all right, though I must admit I feel a bit tired now. Thank you so much, Sarah, for bringing me home and looking after me; you have been so kind and I do appreciate it. Perhaps you will let me go a little way towards repaying you by allowing me to take you out to dinner at the weekend?'

'That would be absolutely lovely, Justin. Thank you very much.'

'I will telephone you one evening this week to arrange it.'

'I shall look forward to that.'

I walked with her to her car and opened the door for her.

'Good night, Justin,' she said and kissed me on the cheek.

Her lips felt soft and as her hair brushed against my face I became aware for the first time that she was wearing a delightful but subtle perfume that seemed uniquely different from anything I had ever smelt before. It was quite enticing and I kissed her on the cheek. For a brief moment we shared what to a casual observer would probably be described as a friendly hug but somehow it seemed a lot more than that to me.

' Goodnight, Sarah, and thank you once again.'

She kissed her fingers, placed them on my lips and then gave me the most beautiful smile as she got into her car.

CHAPTER THIRTY-FIVE

'I simply don't believe it,' I heard Spencer exclaim as I went into his surgery to wish him well for the day.

I felt more or less back to normal after my stay in hospital, though I still had considerable tenderness at the back of my head and a grim determination not to have any further involvement with the general anaesthetic machine.

'I really don't believe it,' Spencer repeated. 'There is absolutely no need for it.'

'Good morning, Spencer,'

'Justin, welcome back, how are you feeling?'

'I'm all right, thank you, Spencer. What's the problem? What don't you believe?'

'It's bureaucracy gone mad. The powers that be have now decided it is necessary to test all X-ray machines in dental practices to ensure they are safe. It's ridiculous. Everyone possessing an X-ray machine is now required to register it with the Department of Radiological Safety and to have it tested on a regular basis to ensure that the machine meets their safety standards. If you ask me, it is simply to find jobs for the boys.'

'So when will they be coming to inspect the machine?'

'That's just it – they won't. Oh no. They have no intention of getting off their big fat backsides and doing some work. They expect us to do it for them. They have sent me some X-ray films, which are labelled 1 to 4 and they want me to expose each of the films with my X-ray machine in a certain way. They want me to expose the first film at the same exposure time as if I were taking an X-ray of an upper incisor and the second film as if I were taking an X-ray of a lower back molar.'

'There's no difference as far as we are concerned. You told me to use the same exposure for everything; upper or lower, front or back.'

'That's right. There is no need to keep fiddling around with the exposure time. We are only talking about fractions of a second, anyway. This whole thing is a complete nonsense. As I said it's bureaucracy gone mad.'

'What do they want you to do with the other films?'

'The third one is to be exposed at 0.1 seconds and the fourth one at 0.3 seconds.'

'It will be well nigh impossible to do that on your machine with any degree of accuracy, because the markings have worn off the scale. You can't see what it's set to.'

'We never have to alter the timer because there isn't any need; we get perfect results with it set as it is.'

'But what exposure time is it set to?'

'I'm not sure. About half a second I think. It might be a bit more.'

'That's a lot more than the 0.1 seconds they are talking about.'

'I don't think you can take any notice of that. The proof of the pudding is in the eating and my experience with my machine over a long period of time has shown me that there is nothing to be gained by adjusting the exposure time. The same setting is fine for everything. It's probably a bit on the generous side but I think it's best that way. If you don't give enough exposure, the films will be too faint to be of any use. It also helps to compensate if the developer is getting a bit stale.'

'So you are saying that exposing these four films is all there is to the test. Is that right?'

'Yes, that's right. Oh, there is one more film. This one has been exposed already at the Department and we have to develop it in the same way as we would one of our own X-rays. That's to check that we are developing our films properly. It's an insult to our intelligence. A chimpanzee could develop an X-ray film – we don't need some boffin checking up on us. I feel like writing a strong letter of complaint saying that I am offended to be told, with all my years of experience, that I am not trusted even to develop an X-ray film.'

'There's no point in getting annoyed about it, Spencer. It's got to be done, so why not just do as they ask and send the films back? After all, we have noticed that the machine is making a strange noise, so this test will put your mind at rest one way or the other as to whether there is anything wrong with it.'

'Don't talk rubbish, Justin. I don't need my mind putting at rest. I've told you there is absolutely nothing wrong with the machine. We get perfect X-rays most of the time. There are bound to be occasions when the results aren't quite as clear as you would like, but there can be many reasons for that. I don't think you can start blaming the machine.'

'It is amazing that they can find out everything they need to know just from five films.'

'Sounds a bit far fetched to me,' scoffed Spencer. 'They say that after examining these films they will be able to provide a comprehensive report on the machine. Can you believe that? It makes me really angry though. I can't bear pointless bureaucracy. My X-ray machine is perfectly all right and there is no need for anybody to question its safety.'

'They obviously think it is necessary to introduce the scheme. After all, an X-ray machine could be dangerous if it's faulty. I suppose they are just doing it to safeguard the public and the operator, who could be irradiating himself and everyone in close proximity without knowing it.'

Spencer clearly did not appreciate my attempt at pragmatism.

'Rubbish. The real reason they are doing it is to make money. Don't think this testing service is free! Oh no! They are charging £20 and there isn't a damn thing I can do about it. The testing is compulsory. It is true I don't have to use *their* service, but if I don't, I have to get the machine tested by someone else within the next three months and send a certificate so I would only be paying someone else, and that might cost more than £20. They know that by offering the test on a plate you are likely to accept it. They've got you over a barrel, in effect, and I see it as daylight robbery.'

At that moment, Ingrid came up the stairs. Spencer heard her footsteps and called out to her.

'Ingrid, will you develop this X-ray film for me?'

'Yes, of course, I will do it as soon as I get a moment. Hello, Justin, how are you feeling? It's nice to see you back at work.'

'I'm not too bad, thanks Ingrid.' I turned to Spencer. 'Don't you think it would be a good idea to change the developer before developing that film? I don't think it has been changed for some time and you wouldn't want the test film to be underdeveloped.'

'The developer is perfectly fine, Justin. I am not going to any extra trouble just to satisfy the bureaucrats. There is no need to change the developer, Ingrid. There is plenty of life left in it yet, and it will be perfectly adequate for the purpose.'

'If you say so, Spencer,' replied Ingrid doubtfully, 'but I too thought it was time we put some fresh developer in the tank; it is very brown in colour.'

'I positively forbid you to change the developer. I have told you it is all right.'

'Whatever you say, Spencer.'

Ingrid and I left Spencer's surgery and I explained to her about the testing of the X-ray machine and how it would be carried out.

'I'm convinced there is something wrong with the machine,' said Ingrid. 'It shouldn't crackle like it does when you take an X-ray. I believe that deep down inside Spencer thinks there might be something wrong with it as well, but he is too stubborn to admit it.'

'Well it looks as if we shall soon know the truth about it. He won't be very happy if he has to pay out to get it repaired at the end of all this. He is blazing mad about having to pay £20 for the test.'

'What do you think about the developer?' Ingrid asked, looking concerned. 'I'm sure it's completely exhausted. It looks like cold tea. I developed a film for him about three days ago and it came out very faint. I can't see the point in failing the test through sheer stubbornness. Shall I put fresh developer in before I develop the test film and not say anything to Spencer?'

'You heard what he said. He forbade you to change it, but I agree with you, I can't see the point in refusing to change the developer when it is obvious that it needs to be changed. My only concern is if we change it without Spencer knowing and the film passes the test, he will then be convinced he is right when he says that the developer lasts much longer than the manufacturers state. You and I both know it should be changed much more frequently than Spencer considers necessary. In any case, he will be very annoyed if he finds out you changed it after he specifically told you not to. I suggest that you drain off a little bit and top it up with fresh solution. That will give it a better chance of working but it will still look fairly brown and it won't be too obvious you have done anything to it if Spencer should look.'

'That sounds a good idea. I will get your surgery ready for your first patient, then I will go and develop the film.'

As it turned out, my first patient failed to keep his appointment. I wasn't surprised because this particular patient, Mr Getting, failed far more appointments than he kept. It was extremely irritating and Spencer had suggested that perhaps we should consider charging him for wasting our time, but so far we hadn't done so.

I was about to settle down in a chair to read the morning paper for ten minutes when Ingrid made me change my plans.

'Will you come and help me to develop this X-ray please Justin? There is a problem with the sun coming through the window.'

I wasn't sure what she meant until I went through to where the X-ray developing machine was situated. It was a very bright morning and the sun was streaming in through the window directly on to the machine.

The machine was basically a light-tight plastic box with the developing solutions inside and there were two leather sleeves through which you put your hands. X-ray film is very much like photographic film and is fogged if exposed to light, and the sleeves were designed to fit closely around your arms to prevent light from reaching the film whilst you were handling it inside the box. Like everything else in Spencer's practice, the developing machine had been in use for a number of years and had been used many times by Spencer himself. The leather sleeves had been somewhat expanded by his arms which were probably twice the diameter of Ingrid's. Consequently when Ingrid used the machine, the sleeves did not fit tightly enough around her arms to be effective in excluding daylight from the X-ray film. On a dull day she could probably get away with it, but she had discovered that when the sun was shining brightly, the film was sometimes ruined by the stray light leaking in around her arms.

'As this is the test film it is vital that I don't mess up the development and I know that if I just go ahead in the usual way, light will get into the developer.'

'So what do you suggest?' I asked, thinking it might be wise to defer developing the film until the sun had moved round.

'I've got a black towel here,' replied Ingrid who had obviously given the problem some consideration. 'If you stand behind me you can wrap the towel round my arms, once I have put them through the sleeves, and then you can hold it tight around them to stop the light getting in.'

It sounded a sensible idea and I did as she suggested. It was unfortunate, however, that Spencer, who seemed to have the knack of appearing at the wrong moment, chose to come into the room just after we had taken up our position. When he saw me standing very, very closely behind Ingrid with my arms round her it was inevitable he was going to jump to conclusions.

'What the hell are you up to now, Justin?'

'It's not how it looks, Spencer.'

'Isn't it? Well tell me how it is, then.'

'We are trying to stop the light from getting into the developing machine.'

'Oh really? I've heard of some lame excuses. Do you expect me to believe that?'

'It's true, Spencer,' Ingrid added with a chuckle. She realised what was going through Spencer's mind and found it amusing.

'I bet it was Justin's idea to do it that way just so that he could grope you.'

'As a matter of fact, it was Ingrid's idea,' I protested.

'Yes, it was my idea,' she confirmed.

Spencer remained unconvinced. 'Ingrid probably suggested it in all innocence. I expect you couldn't wait to get your hands on her. You are going to have to keep your hormones under control, Justin.'

'Spencer, we are trying to ensure that your test X-ray film is developed properly. You want to pass this test, don't you? It won't pass if it's fogged during development. I think it's a brilliant idea of Ingrid's to keep the light out of the machine.'

'Well, maybe,' Spencer agreed reluctantly, 'but I suggest that Ingrid gets Beryl or me to help her next time. I don't think you can be trusted to keep your mind on the job. Anyway, why aren't you with a patient?'

'Because Mr Getting failed to keep his appointment yet again.'

'Damn the man,' Spencer hissed. 'I'm going to charge him for wasting our time. He was my patient for quite a while before you came to the practice, and he was forever failing appointments. I've had enough of it. I'll get Beryl to send him a bill.'

'This is the third appointment he's failed in the last six weeks. He does deserve to be charged.'

'I'll see that Beryl sends it out today. Now. since you have nothing to do you can come and help me expose these test X-ray films.'

We decided that the best way to expose the films was to lay each film flat on a table and point the X-ray beam directly at it from above, but how were we going to alter the exposure time for each film? There were two problems. Because the exposure time was never changed and Spencer's machine had been left at the same setting for many years, the timer had more or less seized up in that position. The knob was virtually impossible to turn and Spencer was understandably reluctant to apply too much force for fear of breaking it. The second problem was that even if it had been possible to turn the knob, the markings on the dial which indicated the exposure time had worn away with age so it was impossible to say what exposure time it was set to.

'How are you going to get round the problem of setting the different exposure times for the four test films?' I asked Spencer.

'I've been thinking about that.'

'And what have you come up with?'

'Justin,' said Spencer switching over to his pompous mode, 'all this business about different exposures in fractions of a second – it's all unnecessarily complicated. I don't believe the people at the Department of Radiological Safety are as clever as they would like us to think they are. I'm not at all convinced they can determine exactly what exposure time has been used.

'So what are you saying? Surely you don't intend using the same exposure on all the films?'

'No. I imagine that they are expecting a range of exposures, but since we can't vary the time we have to do it another way.'

'How do we do that?'

'It's all a question of how much radiation reaches the film. When you take an X-ray, the rays have to pass through the tissues of the body. If there is a lot of muscle, fat or connective tissue in the way, not many X-rays will get through, so you increase the time to compensate.'

'I still don't see how that applies to this test.'

'Justin, you are being very slow on the uptake. All we have to do is to present the Department of Radiological Safety with four films each of which has received a different dose of X-rays. So, the film which should receive 0.4 seconds – i.e. the highest amount of radiation – we expose with the machine set as we always use it. I'm sure that isn't too far away from 0.4 seconds. Then for the next film, we put something in the way to block some of the X-rays.'

'So what are you going to put in the way?'

'Muscle.'

'Muscle?'

'Yes. In the fridge I have some slices of roast ham. I shall lay one slice of ham over the film to block out some of the X-rays. For the third film I shall use two slices of ham and for the fourth film, three slices. That way the amount of radiation reaching each of the films will be reduced incrementally.'

'And you think that will be accurate enough?'

'I don't know, but do you have a better idea?'

'You could get an engineer to look at the X-ray machine and repair the timer for you before you do the test.'

'No. I'm not wasting money like that. In any case, I doubt if it can be repaired. I know how these people operate. They will tell me that the timer needs to be replaced but because of the age of the machine, spares are not available so they will then tell me I have to buy a complete new machine. I've heard it all before and I am not going down that road. Have you any idea how much a new X-ray machine will cost? I can tell you they cost a ridiculous amount of money and modern machines are absolute rubbish anyway. I don't need the timer to work. As far as I am concerned, the machine takes perfectly good X-ray pictures as it is. This test is completely unnecessary, but since it has been forced upon me, I intend to use my ingenuity to get round it as best I can. You set up the first film on the table, point the beam at it and make the exposure. Meanwhile, I will go and fetch the ham.'

CHAPTER THIRTY-SIX

I was quite excited about taking Sarah out to dinner. She was lively, very attractive, sensible, and so far we had got on well together. We seemed to share the same interest in music, literature, our love of the countryside and walking and she was very easy to talk to. I felt relaxed in her company and I think she enjoyed being with me too.

I hadn't heard from Annette since the day she stormed into my cottage. I intended to telephone her at some stage but so far I hadn't got round to it. I suppose, if I was honest, I was a bit apprehensive about doing so as I wasn't sure what sort of reception I would receive. I didn't want to hurt her in any way and I hoped that we could remain friends, but I knew that I didn't share her wish for our relationship to advance beyond friendship. She too was attractive and intelligent, and I enjoyed her company but perhaps the chemistry between us wasn't quite right. On the other hand, I felt that the chemistry between Sarah and I could be right, though it was probably too early to be sure.

I rang her at home, as I had promised, and arranged to take her to The Oak Tree Restaurant at Faringham which was about eight miles away from Luccombury. It was a long-established restaurant with an excellent reputation, though I hadn't been there myself before.

I booked a table for eight o'clock and arranged to pick up Sarah at quarter past seven. She was ready and waiting for me at the door of her house when I arrived. I hadn't seen her in a dress before and she looked sensational. It was well-tailored, just above the knee and its dark green colour looked great with her blonde hair.

'I match your car,' she said as she climbed gracefully into the passenger seat.

'You do,' I agreed, 'but I shouldn't think you want to be described as wearing a British Racing Green dress.'

'I don't see why not; it sounds classy, not at all frumpish. In fact, a bit get-up-and-go. I quite like it.'

'Well, whatever. You look very nice in it, Sarah.'

'Thank you, Justin. How is your head now?'

'It's still a bit sore but much better. I haven't had the stitches out yet so it's still early days. I'm sure it will be fine.'

'That's good. It was a very unpleasant thing you went through. I'm pleased you are getting over it. Now, where are you taking me tonight?'

'I thought we'd try The Oak Tree Restaurant at Faringham. Do you know it?'

'I know of it. I've heard very good reports, but I've never been there.'

'No, neither have I so it will be a new experience for both of us.'

It took us just under a quarter of an hour to make the journey to the restaurant and the first glimpse of it through the trees as we entered the grounds created a very favourable impression. It was built of local stone and dated back to the sixteenth century. It was a rambling sort of building with wings running off the central part in several directions, but it was perfectly proportioned and oozing character. Its setting was magical, surrounded by ancient trees and shrubs which led to a huge area of parkland in the distance. There was a large lawn in front of the restaurant and in the centre of the closely mown grass, dominating the whole picture, was a gigantic oak tree.

'What a magnificent tree,' Sarah exclaimed as soon as she saw it. 'I don't think I've ever seen one as big as that before.'

"It's huge, isn't it? It dwarfs the restaurant and it would make an awful mess of it if it were to fall on it.'

'Don't even think about it. I shouldn't think it will happen this evening though, Justin. There is hardly any wind at all.'

'Well, that's a relief. Are you happy to risk it then?'

'Oh, I think so. I'm starving. We were very busy at work today and I worked through my lunch break.'

The entrance hall to the restaurant was no less impressive than the view outside. It was oak panelled with a big stone fireplace at one end and an oak staircase at the other. There was a small reception desk and a scattering of seventeenth century oak furniture. Although it was quite bright outside, the windows were very small and it was necessary to have the wall lights on but this helped to create a cosier atmosphere.

As soon as we stepped through the door we were greeted by the headwaiter.

'Mr Derwent? Good evening and welcome to the Oak Tree restaurant. Would you like to take a seat in the lounge?'

He led us through to an equally spectacular room with more oak panelling, adorned with oil paintings of country scenes and sumptuous armchairs. We chose to sit by a window which looked out on to distant hills, and ordered drinks whilst we studied the extensive menu.

The choice of food was overwhelming and it was extremely difficult to decide.

'I have never seen such an amazing selection of food,' said Sarah after looking at the menu for some minutes. 'How do you make a selection from all this? I just can't make up my mind. It all sounds absolutely wonderful.'

'I know. It really is an impressive menu. It's a shame we can't try a bit of everything.'

'If you had just a spoonful of each dish there would still be far more than you could possibly eat. Would you mind if I asked you to choose for me, Justin?'

'That's an awful responsibility, Sarah. It would be terrible if I ordered you something you didn't like when there is all this to choose from.'

'I'm sure you won't. I like most things anyway, and I have every confidence that you will know what will be good.'

'All right. As long as you're sure. I won't have the same as you so if you don't like what I order for you, we can always swop.'

I spent quite a while studying the menu whilst Sarah seemed quite happy sipping her drink and looking out of the window. Eventually I was ready to place our order with the waiter.

'For starters I would like to order marinated field mushrooms with warm goats cheese and basil pesto for my friend and monkfish and prawn brochettes on a bed of leeks with a saffron sauce for myself. For main course, seared fillet of salmon on sautéed fennel, spinach and new potatoes with pastis, and, for myself, poached breast of guinea fowl with a sour cream sauce and wild mushrooms.'

'Thank you, sir. And would you like some wine?'

'I would like a bottle of Sauvignon Blanc. That's number 25 on your list.'

'Certainly, sir.'

'That sounds a wonderful choice, Justin,' said Sarah. 'How did you know I adore goats cheese?'

'I didn't, but I had a hunch that you might. Call it intuition if you like. Anyway, I am pleased that I have made a good choice for you.'

'It is so nice of you to bring me here, Justin. It's a wonderful place.'

'I wanted it to be somewhere nice, to thank you for looking after me when I came out of hospital.'

'That was nothing. I was so pleased I got back from Kent in time to be there for you.'

It wasn't long before the waiter called us through to the dining room, which was no less striking than the rest of the restaurant. It was quite a large room created by joining together three smaller rooms. Because of this, it had lots of nooks and crannies and intimate areas and we were led to a table which was hidden from most of the others in the room. Because of its quiet position, it was easy to forget there were other customers in the restaurant and we were able to feel as if the whole of the restaurant and the staff was just ours for the evening.

After the main course we both managed to find just enough room for an excellent crème brûlée. The food was out of this world and the service was impeccable which made it a most memorable meal. After we finished eating we returned to the lounge and the waiter brought us coffee and a delicious selection of mint chocolates. Neither Sarah nor I wanted to leave and we were certainly not put under any pressure to do so by the staff but as we had both reached the point where we couldn't eat another thing and had had as much coffee as we could drink, I asked for the bill.

Settling it was carried out just as efficiently as every other part of the service we had received during the meal and, after thanking the restaurant staff for a most enjoyable evening, we stepped out into the fresh air to drive back to Luccombury.

'Do you want me to drive you straight home, Sarah, or would you like to come back to my cottage and listen to some music?'

'I'd like to come back, Justin, if you don't mind. I am so full it will be lovely just to sit and relax for a while.'

I helped Sarah into my car though she was perfectly capable of getting into it unaided in spite of her tight skirt. She settled into the passenger seat and appeared to have a look of sheer contentment on her face, which pleased me. The more time I spent with her, the more I liked her.

'Do you want more coffee or something else to drink?' I asked her once we were safely back in the sitting room of my cottage.

'I couldn't eat or drink another thing. I just want to sit here quietly and listen to some decent music. Do you have Beethoven's Pastoral Symphony? That would seem to be a suitable choice, bearing in mind that we are in the heart of the country here.'

'Yes I do. I'll put it on. Didn't you live in the country in Kent?'

'We did but it wasn't as quiet as it is here. It was much more built up where we lived. We didn't have to go far to reach open countryside, but that's not quite the same as living in a little country town.'

'I'm glad you like it here, Sarah, and I am very pleased that you decided to leave Kent and come to live here.'

'I'm pleased too.'

As soon as the record started to play Sarah kicked off her shoes and snuggled up close to me on the sofa. I put my arm round her and the smell of her perfume gently wafted over me. It was a lovely, warm, relaxed feeling and I think I could be forgiven for wishing that time would stand still.

Sadly, my reverie was brought to an abrupt end by a loud and insistent banging on my front door.

I immediately thought that it would be Annette. 'Oh no,' I said to myself, 'I really hope it isn't. Sarah and I have had such a lovely evening and a confrontation with Annette would completely spoil it. Please don't let it be her.'

I even wondered if it might be wise to hide Sarah somewhere out of the way but quickly decided against it. She would probably have thought I was being stupid and it wouldn't go down well with her. No, it wouldn't be fair to her either; she was there as my guest and I didn't mind who knew it. Annette would have to accept that I was free to go out with whomever I wanted.

'Who on earth can that be?' I said to Sarah, pretending that I had no idea. I was afraid to open the door but the banging was repeated and it was clear that I wasn't going to be able to ignore it. I was convinced that it had to be Annette and she wasn't going to be at all happy to see Sarah and me together. Slowly and deliberately I went to the door trying to sort out in my mind how I was going to handle the situation. I turned the knob and felt my heart rate increase with apprehension as I pulled the door open.

'Justin, can I come in?'

I can't describe my relief when I saw that it wasn't Annette at the door. It was Ephraim.

'Sorry to disturb 'ee, Justin. I've got somethin' to show 'ee. I'd like some advice on it, like.'

I stepped back to allow Ephraim to enter. He was wearing his rubber boots and looked as if he had just walked through a field of mud, but I was still pleased to see him even though he left a brown trail across the floor. Nellie followed him in, equally as messy. She flopped down on to the carpet in front of the fire and little pools of muddy water dripped off her fur and formed a complete ring around her. Ephraim was carrying a cardboard box.

He looked quite startled when he saw Sarah.

'I didn't realise 'ee were busy,' he said.

'That's all right,' I replied, though now that the anxiety I had felt when I thought Annette had dropped in on me, had passed, I wasn't entirely happy about having my time alone with Sarah disturbed.

'Sarah, this is Ephraim my landlord. Ephraim, my friend Sarah.'

'Delighted to meet 'ee, my dear,' said Ephraim. 'I wouldn't recommend 'ee shake hands wi' I cos I's just been cleanin' out the pigeon loft.'

'Hello Ephraim. I'm pleased to meet you,' Sarah responded, though I noticed she wisely didn't hold out her hand to him.

'I 'as somethin' 'ere I'd like 'ee to look at. What wi' 'ee bein' into teeth and wot 'ave 'ee. I reckons 'ee might knows wot 'tis.'

Ephraim placed the cardboard box very gently on the table.

'It looks very fragile from the way you are handling it,' Sarah remarked as she looked at the filthy state of his hands and felt relieved that she hadn't been put into the situation of having to shake hands with him.

'Aye, 'tis that.' Ephraim confirmed. 'I found it yesterday in wall of fireplace of all places. Must 'ave bin there all these years, see, wi'out I ever knowin' it. Wall's bin steadily crumblin' way fer some time an' I thought that I best do summat 'bout it 'fore it fell down, like. I shifted some stones and this popped out.'

'You mean the fireplace in your cottage?'

'Aye, that's right.'

Ephraim opened the box with the same care as when he had placed the box on the table and withdrew a small animal skull, which was completely intact even to most of the teeth.

'Jake Lawton were wi' me when I found it and 'e thought might be cat, like. But I said 'no, 'taint cat. Teeth's too big for cat.'

'You are right about that, Ephraim. The teeth are too big. It's a strange looking skull, isn't it? I am puzzled by this bony crest along the top of it. What do you think it is?'

'Don't rightly know, Justin. Looks sort o' lizard-like from shape of its head, see, but teeth don't look right for lizard. That's why I've come to ask 'ee. I thought 'ee might just know from teeth, 'ee dealin' wi' teeth like.'

'I *deal*, as you put it, with people's teeth, not animals'. But you are right. The head is shaped like a lizard, but lizards don't have teeth like that. You're a countryman, Ephraim, and you are familiar with most animals. Haven't you any idea?'

'Don't look like anything I ever saw afore.' He looked me squarely in the eye with a slightly self-satisfied expression and continued, 'but I 'as got a thought on the subject.'

'So, what do you think it is, then?'

Ephraim moved in closer and looked around him to as if to see if anyone else was present in the room to hear what he was about to say. He continued to speak in hushed tones.

'I've looked at this 'ere skull long and 'ard and does 'ee know what I thinks 'tis?'

'No, I don't, Ephraim. Go on, tell me.'

There was a long pause. I looked at Sarah who was finding the whole thing highly entertaining and trying desperately not to laugh especially as Ephraim was looking so deadly serious about it.

'As I said 'taint like nothin' I knows. I'll tell 'ee what I thinks 'tis.' Another long pause. 'I thinks 'tis one o' them there dinosaurs.'

The idea seemed more than a bit ridiculous but I didn't want to hurt his feelings so I didn't dismiss the idea out of hand. I had to admit that I didn't know what it was, so how could I pass judgement? Sarah looked very surprised at Ephraim's suggestion.

'It's an interesting thought, Ephraim, but apart from anything else I don't really think it looks old enough. The colour of the bone suggests to me that it is old – very old – but if it were a dinosaur, I think that would make it over two hundred million years old.'

'That old?' Ephraim replied in disbelief. 'That is old, ain't it?'

'I'm fairly sure that's how long ago it is since dinosaurs walked the earth. Is that right, Sarah?'

'I don't know exactly, but yes, I think you are right. They belong to the Mesozoic period, don't they?'

'I see what 'ee means,' said Ephraim. 'Looks a bit too well-preserved like to be that old, don't it? Though 'ee 'as to remember 't'as bin in wall o' fireplace for near on last three hundred years.'

'But that is only a tiny fraction of two hundred million.'

'Aye, suppose 'tis.'

'The other thing to consider is that dinosaurs were, I think mostly herbivorous.'

'What's that?' asked Ephraim.

'They were plant eaters.'

'So? What's that got to do wi' it?'

'Well,' I said trying to sound knowledgeable when, in fact I was very unsure of my ground. 'I am fairly sure that dinosaurs were plant eaters, not meat eaters and the teeth of this animal, whatever it is, look like the teeth of a carnivore – a meat eater.'

'And 'ee can tell that from they teeth? That's clever, that is. I knew 'ee would know summat 'bout it. I said to Jake that 'ee would be the one to ask.'

'I don't think it's true that they were all plant eaters,' Sarah interjected. 'There were lots of different types of dinosaurs which spanned a long period of time. I think some of them were carnivorous.'

'Sarah is probably right, Ephraim, but these teeth are as well formed as a present day dog's. I wouldn't have thought that dinosaurs' teeth were like that, but I could be wrong and I have to say that I honestly don't know what it is.'

'What does 'ee suggest I does to find out 'bout it?'

'Might be worth asking a vet, first of all, to see what he makes of it. He would probably know if it is some present day animal's skull. If he thinks it's ancient then perhaps you need to show it to an archaeologist. A museum might be able to help.'

'I could take it to show Colonel Crowshaw.'

'Is he the vet in Market Square?'

'Aye that's 'im. Bin there years. I 'ad to take Nellie to see 'im once when she 'urt 'er paw, like. But that's the only time. Nellie and vets is bit like me an dentists. We keeps away from 'em.'

Ephraim carefully packed the skull back into its box. 'I shan't detain 'ee any longer, I can see 'ee don't want me 'ere, but I'll let 'ee know how I gets on wi' it. Thanks for 'avin' a look at it.'

With that, he and Nellie made a fresh trail of mud over the cottage floor and back out through the front door.

CHAPTER THIRTY-SEVEN

Sarah and I were once more alone together. I restarted the record player and we took up our position on the sofa again. Sarah snuggled up even closer and I replaced my arm around her and lightly caressed her shoulder. Our heads came closer together and I felt her hair brush my face. The delicate fragrance of her perfume was completely captivating and almost without thinking I gently kissed her cheek. She responded instantly by turning towards me and our lips met. Her kiss was soft and warm and made my senses tingle. We held on to the moment for several seconds and it seemed that neither of us wanted to be the one to bring it to an end. Sadly, the telephone, which was situated only a few feet away from us, suddenly demanded attention by ringing harshly and intrusively. My first reaction was to ignore it but it was difficult to do so when it was so close and so insistent.

Reluctantly I picked up the handset. 'Hello.'

'Hello, Justin, it's Annette here. I'm phoning to apologise to you for my behaviour on Tuesday. I was so upset when I found out that Sarah had picked you up from the hospital because I wanted to be the one to take you home and look after you. You know I have strong feelings for you, Justin, and I was very jealous. I suppose that is why I behaved as I did, but I just couldn't bear to think of you with someone else. I realise now that I overreacted and I believe you when you say that there is nothing between you and Sarah. I am so sorry I doubted you. Can we please forget the whole thing and take up from where we were before it happened?'

'Er … I am afraid… er … this isn't a very good time.' I stammered, breaking out in a cold sweat. I was sure Sarah was close enough to be able to hear Annette's voice.

'Why not?

'I'm rather busy at this moment.'

'You've got someone there with you, haven't you, Justin? It's Sarah isn't it? Isn't it? It is, I know it is.' Annette sounded as if she were becoming slightly hysterical. 'Oh. Justin, you mean, rotten, two-timing, horrible, uncaring, cruel, heartless man! How could you do it to me when you know I love you so much? I would do anything for you and you don't care a fig about me! I hate all men. I thought you were different from the others but I see now that you are just the same. I hate you!'

She slammed the phone down and I am not sure whether I was upset or simply relieved that the conversation was over.

'What on earth was all that about?' asked Sarah who must have heard a good deal of what Annette had said.

'It was Annette.'

'I rather gathered that. What's the matter with her this time?'

'She phoned up to apologise for her outburst on Tuesday, but when she realised you were here she got upset again.'

'What are you going to do about it?'

'I don't see what I can do. I think she is inconsolable and there is nothing I can say to her that will make her feel any differently. I am sorry she's so upset, but I think I shall just have to leave her to get over it.'

'She obviously has strong feelings for you. Are you sure you didn't encourage her at some stage?'

'No, I can assure you I didn't.'

'Well it just seems a bit strange to me that she should feel so deeply involved if, as you say, you have never indicated to her that her feelings were reciprocated.'

'I swear to you that I have never given her any reason to think that I felt anything for her other than friendship. You must believe me, Sarah.'

I am not sure whether she did believe me entirely and the incident certainly cooled any ardour that had been developing between us before Annette's phone call. I didn't somehow consider it appropriate to try to kiss her again though it might

305

have helped to settle her doubts if I had. My failure to rekindle the spark that had been produced between us earlier in the evening was, on reflection, a serious error. Although we held hands and sat closely together on the sofa, there was an underlying element of uncertainty in our relationship and, after about half an hour, Sarah said that she really ought to be getting back home.

Although we chatted for the whole of the journey to her house, our conversation was somehow strained. Neither of us mentioned Annette, but she was clearly very much in both our minds. When we arrived at Sarah's house we exchanged a quick peck on the lips and she thanked me for a lovely evening and said how much she had enjoyed the meal. I wanted to ask her not to let the business with Annette spoil things between us and for an instant I almost took her in my arms and kissed her passionately, but for some reason my courage failed me and I let her go. As I drove back home alone I chastised myself for not trying harder to quell her doubts about Annette and I realised that when it came to dealing with women and romantic relationships I still had a great deal to learn.

CHAPTER THIRTY-EIGHT

I didn't sleep very well that night. I kept thinking about Annette and whether or not I should get in touch with her and try to talk things through. I knew she hadn't fully recovered from her broken engagement and I didn't want to cause her more distress at a time when she was not strong enough to deal with it. She had obviously read far more into our relationship than was justified, but there was no doubt she was very, very upset. Surely she wouldn't do anything stupid, but I couldn't be sure. I would never forgive myself if anything happened to her because of me. I also thought about Sarah. It seemed to me that there was a chance that we might strike up a lasting relationship and I didn't want anything to spoil that possibility.

As I left for work, Ephraim accosted me.

'Good mornin', Justin. I'm glad I caught 'ee before work. I wanted to have a quick word.'

'Good morning, Ephraim. I can't hang around for long; my boss is away on holiday so I am in charge, and I wanted to get to the surgery a bit earlier. What is it you wanted?'

'I've bin thinkin'. If this 'ere skull is dinosaur, will it be worth a lot o' money?'

'I don't really know, Ephraim. How do you put a value on something like that?'

'It's just that if it should be worth somethin', well a little bit extra wouldn't go amiss like, if 'ee sees what I means.'

'Oh I see. You are hoping to sell it, are you?'

'Well, it's bin in my possession so to speak fer a good few year, an' they says that possession be nine tenths o' law, an finders keepers, so I reckons it belongs to I which means that I 'as a right to sell it an' keep the profit.'

'I suppose it does. If it is a dinosaur, a museum might buy it, but I think it is usual for people to donate objects which are of historic interest. After all, it isn't much use to you, is it? Maybe it depends how much money the museum has to spend to buy an item for display and how badly it wants it. They might buy it if they think it is particularly interesting, but it seems to me that most of them are strapped for cash. I honestly don't know the answer. You will have to make some enquiries.'

'Oh, I intends to. I's goin' to see old Colonel Crowshaw this mornin' first off an' see what he says 'bout it. If he thinks it be a dinosaur. I'll most likely take it to Dorchester Museum. If it's as old as you said it would be if it's a dinosaur, then it ought to be worth a pretty penny. Could make me a rich man.'

'I don't know about that, Ephraim. I wouldn't build my hopes up too high if I were you, but I wish you luck with it. Let me know how you get on.'

'I will, bye, Justin.'

Because Spencer was away, my day turned out to be quite hectic, which wasn't a bad thing because it took my mind off Annette and Sarah. I quite liked being in charge of the practice and I wanted to prove to Spencer and myself that I was capable of running it efficiently. Spencer would be in France by now. He had thought of very little else for the past four weeks and an enormous amount of energy had gone into organising it. He was going to the French Alps in his Frazer Nash together with a good many other vintage sports car fanatics. They would be travelling many miles in their old cars but they went in a group and were willing and ready to help each other out in the event of mechanical breakdown. There was obviously a wonderful kindred spirit, which Spencer loved. Every day was rounded off by a sumptuous meal in a top-class restaurant or hotel where food and drink was imbibed in abundance. Spencer realised that he would gain a considerable amount of weight during the two weeks, hence the need for radical dieting beforehand. As usual, however, his will power had not been strong enough to make a significant impact on his steadily increasing plumpness. He was aware that he was almost certain to add more pounds than he had succeeded in losing during his preparation for the holiday.

Once again he told me how much he valued the fact that I would be around to 'hold the fort', as he put it, whilst he was away, and whilst I was quite happy to run the practice on my own I had come to realise that Spencer had a lot of quite difficult patients. It wasn't long before Mr Archibald made his daily visit for a denture ease and just when I thought I had dealt with all the emergencies, another of Spencer's eccentric patients requested my help.

'It's Mrs Fern,' said Beryl. 'Apparently she has had toothache for the past five days and it was so bad last night she couldn't sleep at all. I've put her in with you at the end of this morning's session. Is that all right?'

'Yes, that's fine, Beryl.'

'She is a little bit odd, I have to say. Poor soul lost her husband about five years ago and has never really got over it. She suffered a sort of nervous breakdown and was in a mental hospital for a long time. I think she is still on medication.'

'That's very sad,' said Ingrid.

'Yes, it is,' I agreed. 'I'll look after her, Beryl and see if I can sort out her toothache.'

Mrs Fern arrived twenty minutes early and had quite a long wait because I was running late anyway. Finally, Ingrid showed her into my surgery.

'Do you mind if I leave for lunch now, Justin?' Ingrid asked. 'You know I have arranged to meet a friend who is over here from Germany because I thought we would finish early this morning, but I can phone her and cancel it if you want me to stay here whilst you treat Mrs Fern.'

'No that's all right, Ingrid. Beryl is in the office; I will get her to help me if I need to. You go and enjoy your lunch. I will see you this afternoon.'

'Thank you, Justin, that is very kind of you.'

'Now, Mrs Fern, I hear you have had severe toothache. Would you like to tell me about it?'

'Are you Mr Derwent?'

'Yes, that's right.'

'I wasn't expecting you to be so handsome. You are a nice looking boy, aren't you? I am sure we shall get on well together.'

'When did your toothache start?'

'Sometime last week. You know, I've had awful trouble with my teeth. You wouldn't like to take them all out for me, would you?'

'I'm just covering for Mr Padginton whilst he is on holiday. I can do something with the tooth that's hurting, but as for the others, that's up to Mr Padginton.'

'I've been asking him to take them all out for ages now but he won't do it. I haven't got many upper teeth left – I've got a plate – but he says lower plates are more difficult to wear, so he insists I keep my own teeth at the bottom but they aren't very good and now one of them is giving me jip.'

'It is true that lower dentures are generally difficult to wear. Tell me which tooth is hurting.'

'When I was in hospital lots of people in there didn't bother to wear their false teeth. But I thought they were stupid not to. Do you know there were some very nasty people in there who would steal anything, even your teeth, just to be spiteful? The only safe place for them was in your mouth. Do you know I lost my bra one day and I'm sure it was stolen. It was new you see – a black one from Marks and Spencer. My husband always liked me in black underwear. I was in hospital a long time but I'm much better now. The doctor has halved my tablets. I was on eight a day, but now I only take four.'

'Will you tell me which tooth is hurting, Mrs Fern?'

'Do you know what I really need to put me right?'

'No, Mrs Fern, what's that?'

'A man, that's what I really need. Every woman needs a man, you know, and me more than most, especially on cold nights. It just isn't the same to take a hot water bottle to bed with you.'

'Will you please tell me which tooth is hurting?'

'If only I had a man. I miss my husband you see. It's over five years now since he was taken from me. I had just had my appendix out. Very sudden it was, he was only fifty two, and had never had a day's illness in his life. Just shows you, doesn't it? Now me, I've been in and out of hospital all my life. My belly is just like a road map where I have been opened up. Look, I'll show you.'

'Er, I don't think so, Mrs Fern,' I said backing away as she started unzipping her skirt. 'Please, I really don't want to look.'

I beat a hasty retreat into the office to seek Beryl's assistance.

'She's unzipping her skirt to show me her operation scars, Beryl. Will you please go and ask her to get dressed? Then you had better stay with us whilst I try to carry on with her treatment. Call me in when she is decent.'

I could hear Beryl telling her that she must cover herself up and that I would not go back to treat her teeth unless she promised not to behave improperly. Finally she called me back into the surgery.

'Now, Mrs Fern,' I said beseechingly, 'will you please tell me which tooth is hurting?'

'I think it is all of them, Mr Derwent. I think you will have to take all of them out to stop my pain.'

'But when you came in you said it was just one tooth that was hurting.'

'Well, now I think it is all of them. Would you like to examine me?'

The smile on her face and the look in her eye suggested to me that there was a strong element of *double entendre* as she said it. Beryl was also aware of it.

'Mr Derwent will look at your teeth if you open your mouth for him,' she snapped. Mrs Fern did as she was asked and, in spite of an in-depth investigation, I was unable to establish that any one tooth was worse than the others, though none of them was particularly healthy.

'I think you might have a slight infection,' I declared finally. 'I will give you some antibiotics to tide you over until Mr Padginton gets back, and then you can let him have a look.'

'I don't think I want to see him any more, Mr Derwent. Can't I transfer to you? He is married and you are single. In any case, you are much younger and more handsome. I will come to see you in future.'

I tried to make Mrs Fern understand that she was Mr Padginton's patient and that it was not possible for her to become my patient on a permanent basis, but try as I might I could not get through to her. Beryl tried also but Mrs Fern remained convinced that she would be seeing me for her dental treatment from now on. As she left my surgery clutching her prescription, her final words to me were 'I have heard you do home visits for your special patients. I shall look forward to you coming to me next time.'

CHAPTER THIRTY-NINE

As soon as my last patient had left that afternoon I drove round to Annette's home. I had been worried about her all day. She sounded so upset on the phone and I was genuinely concerned that she might do something irrational. I was, after all, quite fond of her and I cared enough to want to try and help her.

When she came to the door it was obvious she had been crying. 'Can I come in, Annette? I think we need to talk.'

'I don't think there is anything more to be said,' she sobbed. Nevertheless, she stepped aside and let me enter.

'What time did you finish work?' I said, wondering how I was going to handle the situation. My decision to go and see her had been an impulsive one and I hadn't really thought through what I was going to say to her.

'I didn't go to work today. I didn't feel up to it.'

'I'm sorry, Annette. Are you feeling better now?'

'No, I feel terrible. You have hurt me so much, Justin. You don't seem to realise.'

'I never meant to hurt you.'

'Well, you have. I thought we had something special between us, but I see now that I mean nothing to you.'

'That's not true. I greatly value your friendship.'

'I thought we had more than just friendship.'

'I never said to you that we were more than friends.'

'Well, maybe you didn't say it, but you led me to believe there was more.'

'I wasn't aware that I did and I am truly sorry if I gave you the wrong impression. I am fond of you, Annette, but I'm not ready to start a serious relationship with just one person.'

'So what you are saying is that you want to play the field and string lots of girls along all at the same time do you?' scoffed Annette with a hint of venom in her voice.

'No, that isn't what I mean.'

'It sounds like it to me. I think men like you are so selfish. You toy with people's emotions and you don't care who you hurt in the process. You will say anything to talk your way out of a situation without any regard for the truth.'

'That's not fair, Annette.'

'Isn't it? Then why did you lead me to believe there was nothing between you and Sarah and that she had simply given you a lift home from the hospital when in fact you were carrying on with her all the time?'

'I wasn't carrying on with her.'

'I think you were. If it was all innocent between you and she had simply done you a favour as a friend, how is that the very next time I phone you I find that she is with you at your cottage? And it was quite clear that you didn't want to talk to me whilst she was with you.'

'I had taken her out that evening, but that was the only time. I took her out merely to thank her for looking after me when I came out of hospital.'

'I wanted to be the one to look after you when you came out of hospital,' cried Annette, bursting into tears. 'It hurt me so much to find that you preferred to be with someone else.'

'I'm sorry, Annette. It was just the way things turned out. I didn't plan it to happen. Sarah just turned up unexpectedly at the hospital and we went on from there.'

'So where did you take her to thank her for her services?' A hint of malice had crept back into her voice.

'I took her to the Oak Tree Restaurant at Faringham.'

As soon as I said it, floods of tears streamed from her eyes. 'Oh no, not there. It's wonderful there. You must be more than just a bit fond of her to take her there. You have never taken me there; in fact you haven't asked to take me anywhere. How could you be so horrid to me, Justin, when I love you so much?'

She looked at me with a mixture of sadness and anger. and before I could take evasive action she landed a sharp and painful whack with the palm of her hand on my left cheek. 'You deserve that for the way you have treated me.'

I wasn't sure how to respond. The physical assault took me completely by surprise and I felt it was unjustified, as I didn't think I had treated Annette badly in any way. I was sure I hadn't led her to believe there was more between us than friendship; she had just got the wrong impression and blown everything up out of all proportion. It seemed, however, that I wasn't doing a very good job of patching things up between us, and I began to think that if I stayed there talking to her, matters might get even worse. I decided, therefore, to leave.

'I am truly sorry that I have upset you so badly, Annette. I never meant to, and I hope we can remain friends,' I said as I opened the door to go.

'I don't see how we can,' sobbed Annette. 'I don't see how we can,' and she slammed the door shut behind me.

CHAPTER FORTY

It was about six o'clock when I got back to my cottage and I felt absolutely exhausted as well as somewhat shaken by my experience with Annette. I was naturally upset both by the fact that I had made her so unhappy and also because she had felt the need to slap my face which, in my view, was unwarranted. I slumped down on to my sofa, deep in thought, and wondered what I should do next.

One of the disadvantages of living alone, I had found, was that when you arrive home after a hard day, everything will be in exactly the same place as when you left that morning. If you left the house in a mess with unwashed dishes in the sink and books and papers scattered all over the table and chairs they will still be in exactly the same place. It sounds as if this is stating the obvious, but the point I am making is that because you are tired, the mess always tends to look considerably worse than when you left it.

On this occasion, the kitchen looked as if a bomb had hit it because I had been rooting through some books and magazines looking for a particular article on photography. Because I had spent time doing this, I had not had time to wash up after breakfast. The prospect of cleaning up now was not an attractive one and, although I was hungry, it would be difficult to prepare anything to eat until I had done some clearing away. I couldn't make up my mind whether to sit and read, make a cup of tea, pour myself a stiff drink or simply buckle down to sorting out the mess. I was sitting thinking about it when there was a knock on the door. It was Ephraim and Nellie. I wasn't sure whether he was happy or disappointed.

'Hello Ephraim, come in,' I said, though I was in no particular mood at that moment to receive visitors. 'Would you like a whisky?'

'I wouldn't say no, Justin. Thank 'ee kindly.'

I poured him and myself some Scotch and he sat down in my reclining armchair, which was the newest piece of furniture I possessed. I looked at the filthy state of his trousers but said nothing. Nellie lay down on the rug in front of the fire, even though it was not lit.

'I take it you have come to bring me the latest news on the skull. How did you get on?'

'Well, 'tis good news and bad.'

'Are you now a millionaire, Ephraim?'

'Not 'xactly. I went along to Colonel Crowshaw's surgery this mornin'. Don't expect 'ee've ever been, not 'avin' any animals. Do 'ee know 'is receptionist?'

'No, I've not been there. I don't know the Colonel or his receptionist.'

''Ee don't want to neither. Right old cow she be. I got to surgery just after nine this mornin'. Went in there wi' Nellie and she thought I'd brought Nellie to see the vet, like. She says she's probably got fleas and worms and that's what's makin' her bad. She had cheek to tell me I ought to stand outside wi' her so as not to infect other patients, like. Treated me and Nellie as if we were summat she had picked up on sole o' 'er shoe. Looked for all world as if she 'ad bad smell under 'er nose all time. I says to 'er there be nothin' wrong wi' Nellie, I wants to see Colonel Crowshaw that's all, won't take a minute.'

'Did you get to see him?'

'Well, next thing she says is do I 'ave appointment? When I says no, she says 'e's booked up all mornin' unless it's urgent. Then she wants to know 'xactly why I'd taken Nellie there and what was a matter wi' 'er. I said there ain't nothin' the matter wi' 'er, I wants to see vet for summat else. She demands to know what 'twas, but I weren't goin' to tell 'er. I said it's private matter I'd best discuss wi' vet like. She then insists on knowin' if I 'as an animal as needs to be seen by vet. I says well not 'xactly, I just wants to see 'im. You can't see 'im this mornin' she says, 'e's too busy. Says I 'ad to go back at two o'clock when he gets back from

317

'is lunch and 'e'll see I for a few minutes but if 'tain't to do wi' a sick animal 'twould 'ave to be quick. Next she says if Nellie ain't sick not to bring her back wi' I 'cos she don't want 'er spreadin' fleas 'bout the place.'

'So did you get to see the Colonel?'

' Arr. I went back at two and 'e saw me then. Told 'im I'd found a skull and that I'd shown it to a dentist who said it might be dinosaur, an' I wanted 'is opinion on it like.'

'I didn't say it might be a dinosaur, Ephraim. It was you who said that. I said I didn't know what it was, but that I didn't think it was old enough to be a dinosaur.'

'Any road, that's what I said. I thought it might make him take more notice if 'e thought you believed 'twere dinosaur.'

'So what did he say?'

'Took one look at it, laughed and said he were sorry to disappoint I but that it weren't dinosaur's skull – it were a badger's. Then he said he didn't think much to any dentist what couldn't tell difference between a dinosaur an' a badger. Said he wouldn't fancy bein' treated by him in case he got other things mixed up, like. Then 'e wanted to know which dentist 'ad said it.'

'Did you tell him?' I asked somewhat concerned that I had been misquoted so blatantly.

'Oh, arr. I said it were you who 'ad recently come to work wi' Mr Padginton. He said he'd remember to avoid ever lettin' you near 'is teeth. Said it were typical of youngsters of today – not trained properly like they were in old days.'

'Being able to identify the skull of a badger might be important for a vet, but it's not exactly within a dentist's expected field of expertise,' I replied with indignation at Colonel Crowshaw's remarks. 'Anyway, it seems that your skull won't make you a wealthy man after all, then Ephraim.'

''fraid not, but t'weren't a 'total waste o' time 'cos Colonel said 'e knew someb'dy as might want it. Seems this bloke collects skulls and bones an' sort – got quite a collection. Colonel said the skull were well preserved an' 'twere good 'cos it 'ad all its teeth. Gave me 'is address, so off I goes to see 'im straight away. Lives up by Cross Tree Farm in a little cottage there. Do 'ee know it?'

'No, I don't think I have ever been there.'

'Funny place. Bit spooky really. Were full o' stuffed animals. Any road, 'is face lit up as soon as 'e set eyes on the skull. I knew straight away 'e wanted it, like, so I says to I, play yer cards right 'ere, Ephraim old son, and yer could do well. After 'e 'as a real good look at it, 'e asks I how much I wants fer it. I says to him "well, 'tis like this, 'tis summat o' a family heirloom like – bin in family for nigh on three 'undred year, if I did sell it – though I'm not 'tall sure yet whether or not I will – I'd want a tenner fer it.

'Don't think I could run to that,' he says, 'I'll give ee five.'

'Doan' reckon,' I says, ''Ee be worth more 'an that.'

'Six then,' he says.

'Eight,' I says. So finally we settles on seven.'

'That's not bad, Ephraim. Pity it didn't make you a millionaire, but as it didn't cost you anything you can't complain.'

'That's 'ow I sees it. Any road, I just thought I'd let 'ee know. I won't keep 'ee any longer as I 'xpect 'ee got things to do.'

He drained the last drop of whisky from his glass and then lifted the glass higher just to be absolutely certain there was nothing left in it. He put it on the table and shuffled out through the door with Nellie following on at her usual unhurried pace. I poured myself another whisky and sank back into the cushions on the sofa with the chances of my starting to clear up the mess in the kitchen diminishing rapidly. I remained there in a sort of stupor for about ten minutes, then there was another knock at the door. I opened it to find Sarah standing on my doorstep.

'Hello, Sarah, how nice to see you. Are you all right?'

'To be honest, Justin, I'm not very happy,' she replied, stepping into the sitting room.

'Oh dear. Why is that?'

'I'm not very happy because I don't think you have been straight with me.'

'Why do you say that? I don't understand.'

'You haven't been straight with me about Annette. She phoned me up a short time ago and warned me not to get involved with you because you aren't to be trusted. She told me how upset she was because you had let her down so badly. She said that you had led her on into thinking there was something special between you, and then you dumped her to go out with me. She says she thinks you are the sort to make a habit of it, and that I should be on my guard or I will get hurt as well.'

'She said that? But it isn't true.'

'She said that you and she were going out to together seriously and that you had told her that you wanted to be with her and were virtually engaged. She had started to plan your future together and now she suddenly finds that you are seeing me. She is absolutely devastated and has warned me to keep away from you. She thinks you are a womaniser and are the kind of man who will never be faithful to just one girl.'

'I really don't believe what I am hearing. I never led Annette to believe there was anything more than friendship between us. She wanted the relationship to become more serious but I didn't, and I swear that I never said that I wanted us to be together. I think she is deliberately trying to blacken my character in the hope that it will turn you against me.'

'Well then, what's all this about you and she being engaged?'

'There is absolutely no truth in it. We were not engaged.'

'So how do you explain this, then? This morning I went to the hospital to do some physio. I go there occasionally to help out, and I got talking to two of the nurses. We were just chatting generally and one of them asked me how long I had been in the area and whether I knew many people here. I happened to mention that I had just met a dentist who was also new to the area and we had been out together once. She asked me who it was and when I told her it was you she said she thought she knew you. She said if it's the same dentist he was in the hospital last week because he had an accident. I said, "yes, that's right he had to stay in overnight because he cut his head". She then said "that's strange" but when I asked her to explain, she was reluctant to say any more. Finally I managed to get it out of her that whilst you were in hospital your fiancée came to see you. I said that as far as I was aware you aren't engaged and I asked what made her think it was your fiancée. She said that the girl introduced herself as such and that when you were told that your fiancée had come to see you, you didn't say you didn't have one or show any surprise. I asked what she was like and she said she was small with short dark hair and brown eyes, so it was obviously Annette. Apparently you were hugging and kissing each other. The nurse wouldn't lie about it, Justin, so it seems that you have been deceiving me.'

'It's true that Annette came to see me in hospital and said she was my fiancée, but she said that because she arrived after visiting hours and thought that they wouldn't let her in if she said she was just a friend. By saying she was my fiancée she was allowed into the ward.'

'So when the nurse announced that your fiancée had come to see you, I would have thought that the obvious response would be to say that you didn't have a fiancée if that were the case, or at least look surprised. The fact that you didn't speaks volumes, Justin.'

'I did look surprised.'

'The nurse didn't think you did. I know that if someone went around saying they were my fiancé when it wasn't true, I would be very anxious to set the record straight. I am sorry, Justin, but I don't think you have been honest with me, and I don't think you have treated Annette very fairly either. I had hoped that we might be able to build up a relationship, but after this I don't really think I want to see you again.'

I was utterly dumbfounded by what Sarah had said to me. 'Sarah, I swear to you I am telling you the truth. You must believe me. Annette has just read too much into everything. I have never said or done anything to make her think things were serious between us. It is true that I felt sorry for her when I heard she had been jilted, and I tried to be nice to her thinking I was being helpful and supportive and I suppose she has put two and two together and made five. When I realised she wanted more than just friendship I tried to cool things down, but it didn't seem to work.'

'Why didn't you just tell her outright?'

'I tried to, but I was afraid of hurting her because I knew she was vulnerable.'

'Well, it seems that you didn't try hard enough because she was convinced you wanted a serious relationship with her. She said that she now knows that you are the sort of person to string girls along so that you can get your way with them, then you dump them.'

'That's not true. If I were like that then I wouldn't have turned down the opportunity to spend the night with her when she asked me.'

It was the wrong thing to say. A look of horror, disbelief and anger came over her face. 'She asked you to spend the night with her? That proves that your relationship was much more than just friendship, or she wouldn't have asked you.'

'I told you I turned her down. I said ...'

Sarah interrupted before I could say any more. 'You turned her down?' she exclaimed mockingly. 'From what I have just learnt about you I find that hard to believe. I reckon you would have jumped at the chance. What Annette said, now makes sense; she said that your relationship had progressed beyond friendship. Now I know what she meant. I really didn't think you were like that, Justin. It just goes to show that you can't trust anyone. Thank goodness I found out the truth about you before I got more deeply involved. I wouldn't go out with you now if you were the last man on earth.'

Before I could defend myself I received another fierce slap, this time on the right cheek. My front door was slammed with equal ferocity as Sarah stormed out and drove away at high speed.

CHAPTER FORTY-ONE

I was still feeling upset when I went into the practice next morning. My conversations with Annette and Sarah had been going over and over in my mind all night, and I could not believe how things had turned out. I felt that I had been very unjustly treated by both of them and to have had my face slapped twice in the same evening was incredible, yet they were both convinced that I was the villain and had behaved badly. I thought about Tom Cox and Richard Darcy who were obsessed with looking for female companions and I wondered if they had had similar experiences. I decided that if this was what going out with girls was like then I was happy to pursue a life of celibacy.

Ingrid was her usual smiling self when I got to the surgery and greeted me cheerfully. 'Good morning, Justin. It's a nice day at the moment.'

'Yes I suppose it is,' I replied rather grumpily.

'Oh dear, what's the matter with you today?'

'Woman trouble.'

'I'm sorry to hear that. I didn't know you had a girlfriend. You haven't mentioned her. Who is she?'

'There isn't anyone, not anymore. There were two girls on the scene, but unfortunately they each resented the presence of the other one and now there are none.'

'So what you are saying is that you were *two-timing* if that's how you say it in English?' said Ingrid with a twinkle in her eye.

'I wasn't two-timing. I hadn't really dipped my toe in the water with either of them. Anyway, I don't want to talk about it.'

'I don't think I know the expression "dipped my toe in the water",' Ingrid replied.

'I mean that I hadn't started a proper relationship with either of them, and neither of them could really be described as my girlfriend.'

'I must remember the expression. Anyway, Justin, I am sorry to hear that your love life is in turmoil. You can tell me about it if you want to.'

'I don't think I will, thank you, Ingrid. I'd rather forget about it.'

At that moment the postman propelled a bundle of letters through the letterbox and Ingrid went to pick them up.

'This is from the Department of Radiological Safety,' she exclaimed holding up one of the larger envelopes. 'It must be the test results on Spencer's X-ray machine.'

'I'd love to know what it says.'

'So would I. I have a feeling that Spencer is not going to be very happy when he reads it. I am sure there is a lot wrong with the machine.'

Well, it is going to be another week before we find out.'

'Shame,' said Ingrid and a mischievous twinkle returned to her eyes. I could tell what she was thinking and I pre-empted her next suggestion.

'Shall we open it and have a look?'

'We can't, can we? Spencer will be furious,' Ingrid uttered.

'He won't know if we steam it open carefully and then reseal it. In any case, if that confounded machine is dangerous and is firing spurious X-rays at everyone and everything, I think we have a right to know about it as soon as possible because we are the ones who are most at risk from it. I don't particularly want to glow in the dark as a result of using a faulty machine.'

'We haven't got time just now. Your first patient is due any minute.'

'Alright, then we'll open it at lunchtime.'

As soon as we finished morning surgery, Ingrid boiled a kettle of water and I carefully steamed open the envelope.

'I don't believe it,' I proclaimed in utter amazement as I read the letter inside. 'The damn X-ray machine has passed the test. There isn't anything seriously wrong with it.'

'Never in a million years,' gasped Ingrid. 'It can't be all right. The machine is positively ancient, makes terrible noises when you operate it and when you think how Spencer fiddled the test.'

'They have said that the timer isn't accurate, which isn't surprising in view of the fact that Spencer carried out the test by stuffing slices of ham in the way of the beam to reduce the exposure. Also, they say the exposure times need to be adjusted which is simply not possible on that machine, but they haven't said that the machine is unsafe and they haven't said that he can't go on using it. Read the letter for yourself,' I said passing it to her.

'Spencer is going to be impossible when he sees this.'

'I know. He was adamant that the machine was all right and was very pompous about it, but I'm sure that deep down he thought the machine might be seriously faulty, though he would never admit it.'

'Oh well, at least we now know the machine is not dangerous,' sighed Ingrid. 'Give me the envelope and I'll put the letter back and reseal it.'

I hesitated as a roguish thought crossed my mind. 'Supposing we rewrite this letter so that it tells a different story.'

Ingrid immediately guessed what I had in mind. 'That's a very wicked thought Justin and Spencer will go absolutely berserk. Is that what you say in English?'

'It is, Ingrid, but it will be worth it to see his face when he opens the letter next week. Let me take it home to think about it.'

Somehow I had to obtain a sheet of notepaper bearing the heading of the Department of Radiological Safety and it occurred to me that my neighbour living in the other cottage owned and rented out by Ephraim, worked in an office. She eyed me with suspicion when I asked if she had access to a photocopier that would copy the letter heading but leave the page otherwise blank. I had to tell her that we were hoping to play a practical joke on my boss and when she realised it was only intended to be a bit of fun, she agreed to help. The next evening she presented me with several sheets of paper on which I could write my report on Spencer's X-ray machine. Using Beryl's typewriter I wrote as follows:

Dear Mr Padginton

I have serious concerns about the safety of your dental X-ray machine. The recent tests have revealed that it is emitting dangerously high levels of spurious radiation, which are a major health hazard to anyone in the immediate vicinity when the machine is being operated. You must stop using this machine immediately and under no circumstances must you take any more radiographs with it. The defects, which have come to light as a result of the tests, are such that it is quite apparent that the machine could never be rendered safe. We recommend, therefore, that you dispose of it immediately and replace it with a new machine, which complies with the rigorous standards of safety laid down by this department.

Since this machine has obviously been defective for some considerable time, I am naturally concerned about the welfare of all those patients who have had radiographs taken with it recently. I shall be grateful, therefore, if you will furnish me with a list of names and addresses of all patients who have had radiographs taken during the past year. This is a matter of some urgency and I must ask for you to forward this list to me within the next two weeks.

It is my duty to remind you that failure to comply with my recommendations and requests will render you liable to prosecution under the terms of the Radiological Safety Act of 1973.

Yours sincerely

R.N.T. John
Radiological Safety Officer.

'Spencer will go absolutely wild when he reads this,' said Beryl, 'but I do think it will serve him jolly well right, because he didn't know the machine was safe. He knows it has been making strange noises for some time, which could have been an indication that it there was something wrong with it, and yet he couldn't be bothered to get it checked out. He wouldn't have done anything about it if he hadn't been forced to get it tested.'

'It's a great letter,' chuckled Ingrid, ' but it will be difficult to keep a straight face when we watch Spencer read it.'

'I know,' I agreed. 'I don't think I can be there or I'll give the game away.'

'You have to be present to see his face. You can't possibly miss that,' said Ingrid with excitement.

'We'll see. In any case, it is going to be while before Spencer gets back so seal the letter in the envelope and put it with all the other mail he has received.'

CHAPTER FORTY-TWO

'It's good to see you back, Spencer. Did you have a good holiday?'

'Wonderful thank you, Justin. I can't say I am glad to be back though; holidays go so quickly. You look forward to them for so long, and then they are over in a flash. I came back here hoping to ease myself gently back into daily routine but just look at my appointment book. It's positively overflowing with appointments for the entire week. It seems as if half of Dorset have been waiting for me to get back.'

'You shouldn't be such a popular dentist, Spencer. But look at it this way: if you throw yourself into some hard work you will earn enough money to make up for all you have no doubt spent in France.'

'Don't remind me.'

'And how is the weight?' I ventured, thinking that Spencer was looking considerably more portly than when he left home two weeks ago.

'Not too bad,' Spencer replied guiltily then he quickly changed the subject. He started to ask me about how I had coped whilst he was away, but before I had time to answer Beryl interrupted.

'Spencer, Mr Getting has just turned up and would like to see you immediately.'

'Has he come to pay his bill? Can't you deal with it, Beryl?'

'He insists on seeing you.'

'What does he want?'

'I don't know. He wouldn't tell me. He said that he must speak to you personally.'

'Isn't Mr Getting the one who keeps failing appointments?' I enquired suddenly, remembering that he had failed an appointment with me and that Spencer had told me that he did it frequently.

'Yes, that's right. He has failed loads of appointments with me and after the last time when he failed to turn up for you I sent him a bill for £5, partly to cover the wasted time but mainly to show him that we are not prepared to go on having our time wasted. I made it very clear in my letter that we refuse to offer him any more appointments until he has settled this bill. I suppose I had better go and see him but I really don't know why he wants to see me. Why doesn't he just pay up and be done with it? One thing is for sure; I am not prepared to argue about it. I have made the decision and he must pay.'

Spencer disappeared downstairs to the waiting room and I could hear a heated discussion taking place. It was some time before he came back upstairs.

'What a flaming cheek this man has. I can do without this sort of aggravation on my first day back from holiday. It's intolerable. I have never before encountered such downright impertinence.' Spencer's face was bright red and he was clearly in a temper.

'Did you get the money out of him?' I ventured, though it was clear that Spencer's meeting with him had not gone well.

'Don't ask. He has left me speechless.'

'So he didn't pay?'

'No, he didn't. But not only that. He has the sheer audacity, the nerve, the utter impudence to suggest that I owe him money, not the other way round.'

'Really? How does he work that out?'

'That we, or rather I, have wasted his time.'

'And have you?'

'Don't be ridiculous. The man's mad and he's got one hell of a cheek.'

'What is he saying? How is he suggesting you have wasted his time?'

Spencer waved a sheet of paper in the air. 'He presented me with this. It's a list of all his past dental appointments, going back years. He says that I never saw him exactly on time. Sometimes I kept him waiting five minutes past his appointment time, sometimes more than that. He's added it all up and claims that this exceeds the amount of time he has wasted through failed appointments by fifteen minutes. As I was trying to charge him £5 for breaking a half-hour appointment this means that I owe *him* £2.50.'

'It's difficult to argue with that, isn't it?'

'I think he has a confounded nerve to even suggest that I owe him money.'

'So you don't think he has a point?'

'No, I damn well don't. Do you?'

'I can see both sides of the argument. It isn't easy to keep exactly to time and most people realise that. They are prepared to be kept waiting to a degree but we must remember also that they too may be busy people and their time is precious. We expect them to be tolerant when we keep them waiting, so perhaps they have a right to expect a certain amount of tolerance from us too.'

'Come on, Justin, all dentists run a bit late. With the best will in the world, it is inevitable and people generally are prepared to accept it. On the other hand, patients don't have to fail to keep appointments. That can be avoided, and Mr Getting is always failing appointments.'

'According to him, it works both ways and time-wise he is in credit. Anyway, do you intend to pay him £2.50?'

'Not on your life. In the end we agreed to call it straight, but I have warned him that in future he will be charged if he fails an appointment.'

'And you need to make jolly sure that you see him on time.'

CHAPTER FORTY-THREE

'You have had a mountain of mail arrive whilst you have been away, Spencer,' I mentioned casually as I stood by his desk. I tried to see where the envelope from the Department of Radiological Safety sat in the pile but I was unable to spot it.

'I know. It's only when you go away for a week or two that you see how much arrives on a daily basis, though most of it is just junk mail and can go straight in the bin. I have only just started looking at it. It will take me ages to get through it.'

I left him ripping open envelopes and muttering to himself. I would know when he reached the important one because there would undoubtedly be an almighty explosion. I felt sure that if he noticed the name, Department of Radiological Safety, he would hone in on it straightaway.

My first patient arrived and I set about working through my list. Spencer's patients started arriving too so the opening of his correspondence had to be postponed. Ingrid was keeping a close watch on Spencer's activity and she reported to me that he was opening one or two envelopes between each patient, but there was still a huge amount of unopened envelopes on his desk. She decided that she would try to speed up the process. She would wait until he was out of his surgery and then find the envelope and place it nearer to the top of the pile.

About half an hour later she announced to me that Spencer had gone into the office for a cup of coffee and that she had found the envelope and moved it so that there were only two or three envelopes above it. We shouldn't have to wait much longer now.

We didn't have long to wait. As soon as he spotted the label on the envelope he went straight to it. Ingrid was watching through the glass panel in his door and was in no doubt that he was extremely anxious to see the contents. I guess she had probably been right when she said that she thought Spencer was secretly worried about his X-ray machine. From the speed at which he tore open the envelope, it was clear that he was in a hurry to find out the results of the test.

The response wasn't quite as we had predicted. There was no violent outburst and no display of anger. His initial reaction was one of stunned silence. Beryl was in his surgery with him when he opened the envelope and she saw the colour drain from his face. The suntan from his holiday changed instantly from a golden brown to a pale ashen hue, and there was a look of deep concern in his eyes.

'Oh my God,' he cried out holding his forehead with his left hand, whilst his right hand which was holding the letter began to tremble. 'This is terrible, terrible,' he moaned.

'What's the matter,' Beryl inquired, trying desperately hard to avoid giving the game away by laughing.

'It's my X-ray machine. It's worse than I thought. They tell me it's dangerous and that I must stop using it immediately. I shall be in serious trouble if I carry on taking X-rays with it now that I know it is unsafe. What am I to do? We can't manage without an X-ray machine. Oh dear, oh dear.'

Beryl was on the point of bursting into laughter but managed to hide it by pretending to have a sudden coughing attack. She covered her face with her handkerchief and made a swift exit from the room.

Ingrid and I were in the office and Beryl joined us. We all realised that it was going to be extremely difficult to keep up the pretence for very long. One of us would be sure to give the game away. I felt that I had to avoid meeting Spencer face to face.

The office door crashed open and Spencer came in, ignoring the three of us. He picked up the telephone and dialled the local dental supply company.

'Hello, Spencer Padginton of Fothergill House, Luccombury speaking. Can you tell me how much a new X-ray machine will cost?'

'What? How much? Don't you have anything cheaper than that?'

Spencer sank into a chair and beads of perspiration appeared on his brow.

'I've no choice. I shall have to order one. Yes, yes. Get it to me as soon as you can. Next week? If that's the best you can do, it will have to be all right.'

He put the phone down looking completely deflated.

'I should have listened when you said there was something wrong with the machine. Beryl, will you go through all the records and make a list of all patients who have had X-rays taken in the past year? I know it's a huge job, but I'm afraid it has to be done. I have learnt a very hard lesson from all this. From now on, I shall make sure that all the surgery equipment is up to scratch and replace anything that is getting old and worn out.'

'Can we have that in writing, Spencer?' I said smiling.

'Why are you smiling, Justin? I don't think there is anything to smile about. I have just been on holiday for two weeks which cost me a small fortune, and on my first day back at work I discover I am going to have to buy a new X-ray machine at a cost of nearly five hundred pounds.'

I tried hard to control my smile but instead of it diminishing it increased to a faint laugh. It was enough to raise suspicions in Spencer's mind especially when Ingrid's face started to crack as well.

'What's going on?' he demanded. 'Is there some sort of joke going on here that I am not party to? There is, isn't there? What is it? What are you up to?'

Beryl was the one to put Spencer out of his misery.

'The report on your X-ray machine wasn't from the Department of Radiological Safety – we, or rather Justin, wrote it. The real report came whilst you were away on holiday and we couldn't resist opening it to find out whether or not your machine was unsafe. We couldn't believe it when the report said there was nothing much wrong with it and that it had more or less passed the test with flying colours. Justin decided that he would play a trick on you and write a different report on your machine.'

Spencer didn't quite know whether to be overjoyed and hug the three of us or to be furious with us for causing him such anguish.

'Passed with flying colours?' he said beaming from ear to ear. 'I told you there was nothing wrong with it.'

'Not quite with flying colours,' I interjected. 'Here is the actual letter from the Department of Radiological Safety. Although they didn't say that the machine was unsafe, they said that the exposure times needed to be adjusted and that the timer needed to be re-calibrated because the settings weren't accurate. 'Mere details, Justin. The important thing is that the machine is alright.'

'Well, it isn't really all right, Spencer. It might not be unsafe to use, but you can't really say it's all right. You fiddled the test. The timer is seized up and can't be adjusted, so there is no way we can alter the exposures as they request. We can hardly use slices of ham to reduce the exposure when we take X-rays on patients. But anyway, that doesn't matter now because you have ordered a new machine, so we can throw the old one away.'

'What?' Spencer exclaimed. 'I'm not throwing the machine away when there is nothing wrong with it. I shall get on to the dental supply company immediately and cancel the order for the new machine. And you, Justin Derwent, had better watch out because I intend to get even with you for playing a trick like that on me.'